Biological Signals and Receptors

Founded 1992 as 'Biological Signals'

KARGER

Printed in Switzerland on acid-free paper by Reinhardt Druck, Basel

Appears bimonthly: 1 volume per year (6 issues)

Guidelines for Authors

Biological Signals and Receptors

Submission

Only original papers written in English are considered and should be sent to:

Dr. S.F. Pang
Department of Physiology
Faculty of Medicine
University of Hong Kong
Li Shu Fan Building
5, Sassoon Road
Hong Kong
Tel. 852-2819-9260
Fax 852-2855-9730

Peter A. Ward, MD
Department of Pathology
The University of Michigan
Medical School
1301 Catherine Road
Ann Arbor, MI 48109-0602
USA
Tel. 1-313-763-6384
Fax 1-313-763-4782

Daniel P. Cardinali, MD
Departamento de Fisiologia
Facultad de Medicina
Universidad de Buenos Aires
Paraguay 2155 7° Piso
CP 1121 Buenos Aires
Argentina
Tel. 54-1-961-9866
Fax 54-1-963-6287

Manuscripts should be submitted in quadruplicate (with four sets of illustrations of which one is an original), typewritten double-spaced on one side of the paper, with a wide margin. Names and addresses of four experts in the appropriate area of research should accompany each manuscript. Selected scientist(s) will be invited to act as referee(s).

Conditions

All manuscripts are subject to editorial review. Manuscripts are received with the explicit understanding that they are not under simultaneous consideration by any other publication. Submission of an article for publication implies the transfer of the copyright from the author to the publisher upon acceptance. Accepted papers become the permanent property of 'Biological Signals and Receptors' and may not be reproduced by any means, in whole or in part, without the written consent of the publisher. It is the author's responsibility to obtain permission to reproduce illustrations, tables, etc. from other publications.

Arrangement

Title page: The first page of each paper should indicate the title (main title underlined), the authors' names, and the institute where the work was conducted. A short title for use as running head as well as the full address of the author to whom correspondence should be sent are also required.

Full address: The exact postal address complete with postal code must be given at the bottom of the title page. Please also supply phone and fax numbers, as well as your e-mail address.

Key words: For indexing purposes, a list of 3–10 key words in English is essential.

Abstract: Each paper needs an abstract of up to 10 lines.

Small type: Paragraphs which can or must be set in smaller type (case histories, test methods, etc.) should be indicated with a 'p' (petit) in the margin on the left-hand side.

Footnotes: Avoid footnotes. When essential, they are numbered consecutively and typed at the foot of the appropriate page.

Tables and illustrations: Tables and illustrations (both numbered in Arabic numerals) should be prepared on separate sheets. Tables require a heading and figures a legend, also prepared on a separate sheet. For the reproduction of illustrations, only good drawings and original photographs can be accepted; negatives or photocopies cannot be used. Due to technical reasons, figures with a screen background should not be submitted. When possible, group several illustrations on one block for reproduction (max. size 144 × 196 mm) or provide crop marks. On the back of each illustration, indicate its number, the author's name, and 'top' with a soft pencil.

Color illustrations: Up to 6 color illustrations per page can be integrated with the text at the reduced price of CHF 660.–/ USD 545.00 per page. Color illustrations are reproduced at the author's expense.

References: In the text identify references by Arabic numerals [in square brackets]. Material submitted for publication but not yet accepted should be noted as 'unpublished data' and not be included in the reference list. The list of references should include only those publications which are cited in the text. Do not alphabetize; number references in the order in which they are first mentioned in the text. The surnames of the authors followed by initials should be given. There should be no punctuation other than a comma to separate the authors. Cite all authors, 'et al' is not sufficient. Abbreviate journal names according to the Index Medicus system. (Also see International Committee of Medical Journal Editors: Uniform requirements for manuscripts submitted to biomedical journals. N Engl J Med 1997;336:309–315.)

Examples

(a) Papers published in periodicals: Sun J, Koto H, Chung KF: Interaction of ozone and allergen challenges on bronchial responsiveness and inflammation in sensitised guinea pigs. Int Arch Allergy Immunol 1997;112:191–195.

(b) Monographs: Matthews DE, Farewell VT: Using and Understanding Medical Statistics, ed 3, revised. Basel, Karger, 1996.

(c) Edited books: Parren PWHI, Burton DR: Antibodies against HIV-1 from phage display libraries: Mapping of an immune response and progress towards antiviral immunotherapy; in Capra JD (ed): Antibody Engineering. Chem Immunol. Basel, Karger, 1997, vol 65, pp 18–56.

Galley proofs

Unless indicated otherwise, galley proofs are sent to the first-named author and should be returned with the least possible delay. Alterations made in galley proofs, other than the correction of printer's errors, are charged to the author. No page proofs are supplied.

Reprints

Order forms and a price list are sent with the galley proofs. Orders submitted after the issue is printed are subject to considerably higher prices.

KARGER

Fax +41 61 306 12 34
E-Mail karger@karger.ch
www.karger.com

The Guidelines for Authors are available at:
www.karger.com/journals/bsi/bsi_gl.htm

General Information

Biological Signals and Receptors

Publication data: Volume 8, 1999 of 'Biological Signals and Receptors' appears with 6 issues.

Subscription rates: Subscriptions run for a full calendar year. Prices are given per volume.
Personal subscription:
Subscription + postage and handling
CHF 178.85 + CHF 23.50 Europe
CHF 178.85 + CHF 35.50 Overseas
USD 136.85 + USD 23.50
(Must be in the name of, billed to, and paid by an individual. Order must be marked 'personal subscription'.)
Institutional subscription:
Subscription + postage and handling
CHF 511.– + CHF 29.40 Europe
CHF 511.– + CHF 44.40 Overseas
USD 391.00 + USD 29.40
Airmail postage: CHF 36.–, USD 30.00.
(Extra per volume.)

Microforms: Please direct all enquiries and orders to: University Microfilms Inc.
300 North Zeeb Road, P.O. Box 1346
Ann Arbor, MI 48106-1346 (USA)

Advertising: Correspondence and rate requests should be addressed to the Publisher.

Subscription orders: Orders can be placed at agencies, bookstores, directly with the
Publisher S. Karger AG, P.O. Box,
CH–4009 Basel (Switzerland)
or with any of the following distributors:
Deutschland: S. Karger GmbH, Postfach
D–79095 Freiburg
France: Librairie Luginbühl
36, bd de Latour-Maubourg
F–75007 Paris
Great Britain, Ireland: S. Karger Publishers
58 Grove Hill Road
Tunbridge Wells, Kent TN1 1SP
USA: S. Karger Publishers, Inc.
26 West Avon Road, P.O. Box 529
Farmington, CT 06085
India, Bangladesh, Sri Lanka:
S. Karger India Subscription Agency
B–5/132 Safdarjung Enclave
New Delhi-110029
Japan: Katakura Libri, Inc.
2F, Marushima Bldg,
4-6-17 Yushima, Bunkyo-ku,
Tokyo 113-0034

Change of address: Both old and new address should be sent to the subscription source.

Single issues and back volumes: Information can be obtained through the Publisher.

Bibliographic indices: This journal is regularly listed in bibliographic services.

Copying: This journal has been registered with the Copyright Clearance Center (CCC), as indicated by the code appearing on the first page of each article.
For readers in the US, this code signals consent for copying of articles for personal or internal use, or for the personal or internal use of specific clients, provided that the stated fee is paid per copy directly to
Copyright Clearance Center Inc.
222 Rosewood Drive
Danvers, MA 01923 (USA).
A copy of the first page of the article must accompany payment. Consent does not extend to copying for general distribution, for promotion, for creating new works, or for resale. In these cases, specific written permission must be obtained from the copyright owner,
S. Karger AG, P.O. Box,
CH–4009 Basel (Switzerland).

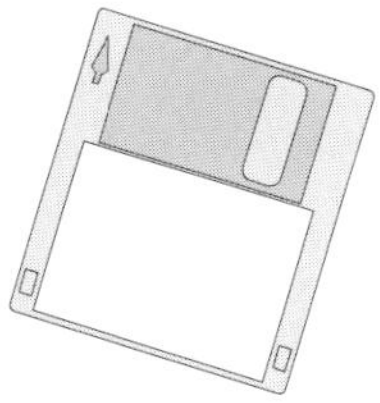

Disk Submission

A **comprehensive version** of these guidelines for the **submission of manuscripts and illustrations on disk** can be accessed online under **www.karger.com/journals/disksub.htm** or requested as a leaflet from the editorial department.

Please follow the general rules on style and arrangement in the **"Guidelines for Authors"** of the journal. Submit a **double-spaced printout** of your manuscript matching the file on disk exactly.

Technical Information

Store only data pertinent to this manuscript. Include your fonts (screen and printer fonts for Macintosh).
For a **text only** manuscript, use a 3.5 inch disk. For **text and illustrations,** use 3.5 or 5.25 Magneto Optical Disc; CD-ROM (DOS or hybrid); iomage Zip/DOS (100 MB), or 44 MB, 88 MB or 200 MB SyQuest. Compress extensive data using ZIP format.

Data Description

Label your disk with the **title of the journal or book** for which it is submitted; a **short version** of the paper's title; your **name,** postal and e-mail adress, fax and phone number; **hard and software** used, including the version; and the **complete list of the file names.** File names consist of eight characters before the dot identifying the file and three characters after the dot identifying the application.

Text and Format

The **preferred word-processing package is MS-Word.** Other commonly used PC text programs and ASCII formats are accepted.
Update your data when you revise subsequent to the reviewer's or editor's decision and mark revisions clearly. Manuscripts accepted for publication are subject to **copy editing:** changes and/or questions will be marked in the manuscript, which will be returned to you with your disk and the galley proofs for checking.
Enter your text continuously flush left. Do not use any layout functions. Do not split words at the end of a line. **Do not use indentations.** Use a blank line before and a hard return at the end of paragraphs. **Arrange headings flush left.** Insert only **one space after punctuation marks.** Insert Greek letters, mathematical symbols etc. with your word-processing program. Use **boldface and italics** as well as sub- and superscript where appropriate. **Tables are part of the text** and should be placed at the end of the text file. Separate the individual parts of a table by lines. Use the tabulator instead of spaces. Format operation data on one line in the same column. **Legends to illustrations are part of the text** and should also be listed at the end of the text file.

Illustrations

Store illustrations as separate files: do not embed them in your text. Export **line drawings/vector graphics** as TIF, EPS or WMF format. Use Photoshop for processing and retouching **scanned half-tone images.** Save the original scan and the processed version. Export **black and white or color images** as TIF or EPS format in their anticipated size in print.
For detailed information on how to submit illustration data on disk please consult the leaflet or **www.karger.com/journals/disksub.htm.**

KARGER

KI 98 DISK

Fax+ 41 61 306 12 34
E-Mail karger@karger.ch
www.karger.com

The Journal Home Page is available at:
www.karger.com/journals/bsi

Biological Signals and Receptors

Hypoxia and Its Preconditioning

Guest Editor

Guo-Wei Lu, Beijing

30 figures, 3 in color, 17 tables, 1999

KARGER

Basel · Freiburg · Paris · London · New York · New Delhi · Bangkok · Singapore · Tokyo · Sydney

S. Karger
Medical and Scientific Publishers
Basel · Freiburg · Paris · London
New York · New Delhi · Bangkok
Singapore · Tokyo · Sydney

Drug Dosage
The authors and the publisher have exerted every effort to ensure that drug selection and dosage set forth in this text are in accord with current recommendations and practice at the time of publication. However, in view of ongoing research, changes in government regulations, and the constant flow of information relating to drug therapy and drug reactions, the reader is urged to check the package insert for each drug for any change in indications and dosage and for added warnings and precautions. This is particularly important when the recommended agent is a new and/or infrequently employed drug.

Printed in Switzerland on acid-free paper by
Reinhardt Druck, Basel
ISBN 3–8055–6963–7

KARGER

Fax+ 41 61 306 12 34
E-Mail karger@karger.ch
www.karger.com

Vol. 8, No. 4–5, 1999

Biological Signals and Receptors

Contents

KARGER

Fax+ 41 61 306 12 34
E-Mail karger@karger.ch
www.karger.com

Access to full text and tables of contents, including tentative ones for forthcoming issues:
www.karger.com/journals/bsi/bsi_bk.htm

Biological Signals and Receptors

Biol Signals Recept 1999;8:247–255

Received: October 10, 1998
Accepted: October 24, 1998

Acute Adaptation of Mice to Hypoxic Hypoxia

Guo-Wei Lu[a] Ding-Wu Ding[b] Mei-Tang Shi[a]

Departments of [a]Neurobiology and [b]Pathophysiology, Capital University of Medical Sciences, Beijing, China

Key Words

Hypoxic preconditioning · Autoprogressive hypoxia · Hypoxic tolerance in vivo · Hypoxic tolerance in vitro · Antihypoxic factor(s)

Abstract

Tolerance to hypoxia in vivo and in vitro was significantly increased by acute and repetitive exposure of mice to autoprogressive hypoxia. The average tolerance times of the successive 2nd, 3rd, 4th and 5th runs of exposure were, respectively, 2, 4, 6 and 8 times as long as that of the first exposure. The survival times under hypobaric chamber and cyanide toxification in the 4th exposure were, respectively, 10 (and even as much as 86) and 4 times those in control mice without exposure to hypoxia. Mandibular respiration and spinal reflex in vitro in hypoxia-resistant animals lasted 5–6 times as long as in control animals not previously exposed to hypoxia. Animals that received brain homogenate from hypoxia-resistant mice remained alive in a hypobaric chamber 2 times as long as those that received homogenate from controls and those that received saline. These results indicate that a kind of quickly developing adaptation with increased tolerance is achieved by acute and repetitive exposure of mice to progressive autohypoxia and some plastic or adaptive changes occur in the brain of hypoxia-resistant animals, including the production of some kind of water-soluble antihypoxic factors.

Hypoxia is an important problem from both a basic science and a clinical point of view, although a large amount of data has accumulated over a century or more, a clear mechanistic understanding of the action of hypoxia and in particular adaptation to hypoxia is still elusive. Vertebrates characteristically do not resist prolonged hypoxia, comparatively few are able to withstand severe hypoxia and almost none can survive chronic anoxia [1]. Previously, large animals were mainly used to study response to hypoxia [2].

KARGER

Fax + 41 61 306 12 34
E-Mail karger@karger.ch
www.karger.com

1422–4933/99/0085–0247$17.50/0

Accessible online at:
http://BioMedNet.com/karger

Guo Wei Lu
Department of Neurobiology
Capital University of Medical Sciences
You An Men Wai Street
Beijing 100054 (China)

The rat has been used to study adaptation to hypoxia experimentally [3, 4]. Adaptation to hypoxia has been investigated to understand acclimatization to high altitude, as well as the effect of chronic hypoxia. Little is known, however, about acute adaptation to hypoxia. It has been reported that tolerance to hypoxia could be achieved by preexposure to 'altitude' for 2 h, or by preprogressive hypoxia for only 3 min [5, 6]. Preexposure of brain slices to hypoxia in vitro for 5 min could also lead to increased tolerance to hypoxia [7].

The brain requires a continuous supply of oxygen and glucose to maintain its viability and function. Mechanisms allowing the brain to survive hypoxia are key adaptations for hypoxic tolerance. The mammalian brain is most vulnerable to oxygen deprivation and thus has been one of the major subjects of intensive study for a long time [1]. Attention has been paid to the activity of isolated mammalian brain, and to the response of in vitro brain slice preparations to hypoxia [8, 9]. No data are available, however, on the change that follows that adaptation through repetitive exposures.

The present work was thus aimed at the following: showing a way to develop tolerance to hypoxia through acutely repeated and progressive autohypoxia in vivo in mice; investigating changes in residual activity of the nervous system after repetitive exposure to hypoxia, and at investigating the effect of brain extract from hypoxia-resistant animals on tolerance to hypoxia.

Methods

Animal Model

Experiments were conducted at room temperature (18–22 °C) on 214 adult BALB/C and Kunming (KM) mice of both sexes, weighing 16.0–22.0 g. The animals were placed into a 125-ml jar with fresh air which was sealed with a rubber plug. The animal was removed from the jar as soon as gasping breath appeared and was switched to another fresh air jar of similar volume within 30 s which was immediately hermetically sealed again. This procedure was repeated 4 or 5 times.

Tolerance Time

The appearance of gasping was regarded as the tolerance limit in each trial. The time period between the beginning of airtightness and the appearance of the first gasping was termed 'original duration of tolerance' for each run. The standard tolerance duration in a standard jar with an effective fresh air volume of 100 ml was calculated as follows:

$$
\begin{aligned}
T &= (T_0/V_e) \times 100 \\
&= [(t_1 - t_0)/(V_0 - V_a)] \times 100 \\
&= [(t_1 - t_0)/(V_0 - W_a/d_a)] \times 100 \\
&= [(t_1 - t_0)/(V_0 - W_a/0.94)] \times 100
\end{aligned}
$$

Where T is the standard tolerance time (min), T_0 is the original tolerance time (min), t_0 is the starting time of sealing, t_1 is the ending time of sealing; V_e is the effective jar volume (ml), V_0 is the original jar volume (ml), V_a is the animal's volume (ml); W_a is the animal's body weight (g), and d_a is the animal's density determined from displacement V_a and measured weight. The average d_a was 0.94, ranging from 0.92 to 1.00.

Hypobaric Chamber and Cyanide Test

Normal mice without exposure to hypoxia were matched for body weight with mice repeatedly exposed to hypoxia. They were put together into a constant low-pressure chamber with PO_2 2.7 kPa (20 mm Hg), immediately after the end of the 4th run, and their survival times were recorded. The other groups, similarly matched, were intraperitoneally injected with lethal doses of potassum cyanide (50 mg/kg) immediately after the conclusion of the 4th run, and their survival times were measured.

Residual Activity

The animals were decapitated immediately after the 5th exposure. The isolated head's jaw movement was recorded by a kymograph and its stop was determined as survival time of the medulla ablongata [10]. The stop of limb movement response to pinch of limb was measured as survival time of the spinal cord [11].

Antihypoxic Action

The brains of normal and hypoxia-resistant mice were removed, weighed, placed into homogenate tubes filled with precooled normal saline and homogenized with an ultrasound cell destructor. The homogenate was then transferred into centrifuge tubes, centrifuged at 4,000 rpm for 5 min, and the supernatant taken.

The other group of animals was randomly divided into three subgroups: intraperitoneal injection of 1.0 ml normal saline, 1.0 ml supernatant (g wet weight/2.5 ml normal saline) from normal animals' brains, and 1.0 ml supernatant (g wet weight/2.5 ml normal saline) from hypoxia-resistant animals' brains. Survival time of these animals was then immediately measured in a hypobaric chamber (PO_2 2.7 kPa or 20 mm Hg) following the injection.

Data Analysis

ANOVA and a paired t test from the SYSTAT program were used for analysis of experimental data. A level of 0.05 or less was accepted as indicative of significance.

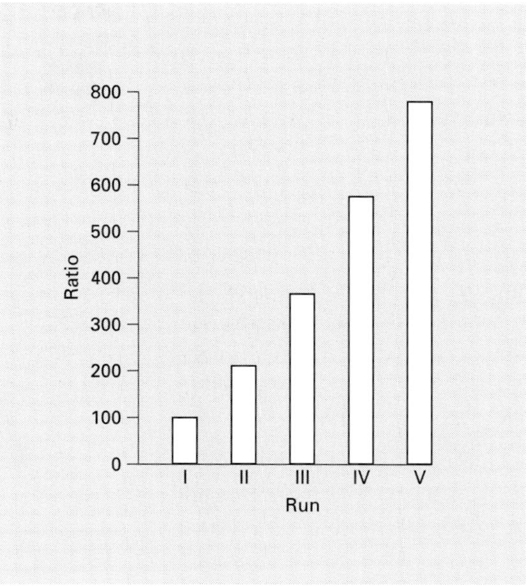

Fig. 1. Tolerance time in different exposure runs. The tolerance time of the first run is normalized at 100.

Results

Overall Behavior

During the first run, the animal's respiration gradually quickened, cyanosis gradually increased and finally spasm-like activity and gasping appeared. A similar behavior was evident during the second run. Starting with the 3rd run, the animal remained quiet most of the time and its respiration became slow, deep, and regular in pattern. Cyanosis became more apparent than before and the eyeballs showed a black-violet color. This seemed to be based on the general state that the animal's life activity gradually and progressively decreasing to a low but stable level.

Tolerance Time

The increment of each run was approximately in an arithmetic progression. The tolerance time of each run lasted significantly longer and longer as the exposure run increased. The average tolerance times of runs I, II, III, IV and V were 12.2 ± 0.31, 25.1 ± 1.03, 44.8 ± 2.72, 71.1 ± 4.49, and 95.5 ± 5.85 (X ± SE), respectively. The tolerance times of runs II, III, IV and V were respectively 2, 4, 6 and 8 times as long as that of the first run (fig. 1). The increase in average tolerance time of animals weighing 16.0–16.9 g was significantly ($p < 0.05$) longer than that of animals weighing more than 17.0 g (fig. 2), suggesting a longer tolerance for the younger animals. One animal in the lower weight group could tolerate airlessness for 232 min in the 5th run, 19 times the tolerance time in the first run.

Survival Time in a Hypobaric Chamber

Normal animals in the control group (n = 15) survived for only 1.60 ± 0.36 min in the hypobaric chamber with PO_2 at 2.7 kPa. However, the animals (n = 15) exposed to hypoxia for 4 runs survived as long as 15.33 ± 2.94 min, almost 10 times the control survival ($p < 0.001$). A few animals in the exposure group survived for 50 min.

As shown in table 1, the normal partners in the pair-matched group survived for only

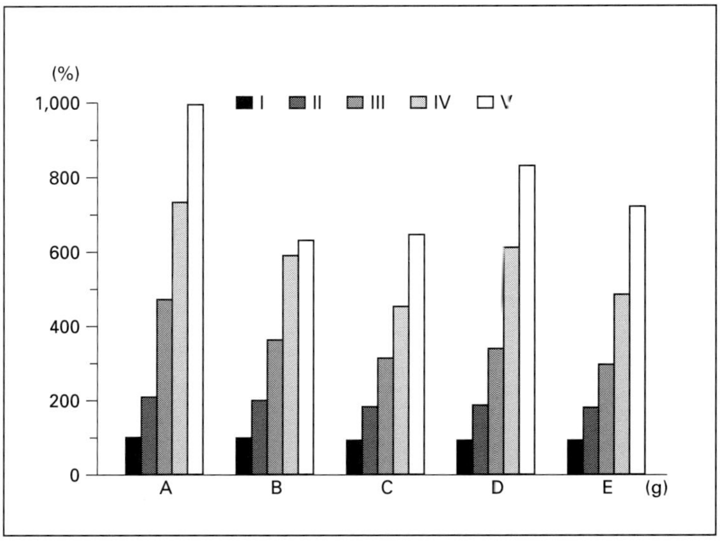

Fig. 2. Tolerance time increment in relation to body weight. The tolerance time of the first run is normalized at 100. Ordinate: percentage change of tolerance time; abscissa: animals' body weight. A = 16.0–16.9 g; B = 17.0–17.9 g; C = 18.0–18.9 g; D = 19.0–19.9 g, and E = 20.0–22.0 g.

Table 1. Survival time (min) under low PO_2 chamber (2.7 kPa, 40 mm Hg) in pair-matched animals

	1	2	3	4	5
Hypoxia exposure for 4 runs	126.0 (20.2)	166.0 (17.5)	71.0 (18.9)	185.0 (19.9)[1]	182.0 (16.2)
Normal controls without exposure to hypoxia	3.0 (19.0)	2.0 (17.5)	0.9 (18.7)	1.6 (19.5)	1.2 (15.4)

Values in parentheses are body weight in grams.

[1] The animal that survived for 185 min was removed from the jar and put into a cage to assess the effect of exposure to 4 runs of hypoxia.

Table 2. Phase and duration (s, $\bar{x} \pm$ SD) of mandibular respiration movement following decapitation

	Apnea			Breathing		
	total	phase I	phase II	total	phase I	phase II
Control (C)	2.7±0.59	0.5±0.16	2.4±0.31	21.9±1.2	6.4±1.00	15.5±1.5
Experimental (E)	41.7±3.57***	19.1±7.47***	22.6±6.07***	82.3±12.4***	10.0±2.16	72.3±12.3***
E/C	15.4	38.2	9.4	3.76	1.6	4.7

*** $p < 0.001$, compared with controls.

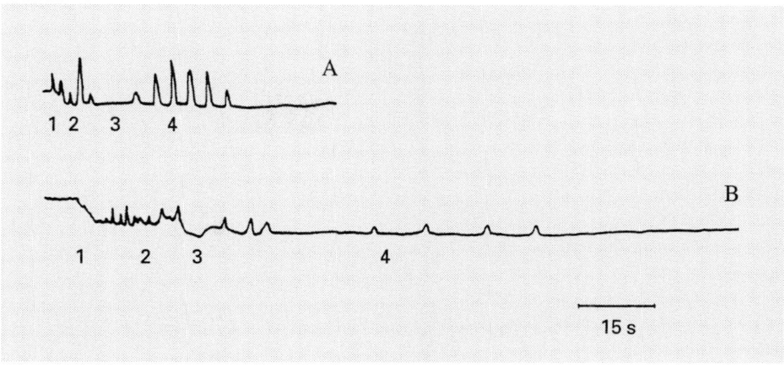

Fig. 3. Mandibular respiratory movement recorded from isolated head. Curve A: recorded from normal animal's isolated head; curve B: recorded from hypoxia-tolerant animal's isolated head; 1, 2, 3 and 4 denote, respectively, phase I apnea, phase I breathing, phase II apnea, and phase III breathing. Note the difference between A and B.

1.7 min in average in the low PO_2 chamber and the repeatedly hypoxia-exposed animals survived for 146.0 min in average, 86 times as long as their normal partners ($p < 0.001$). Mouse 4 in the hypoxia-exposed group survived for 185 min and was healthy the next day.

Survival Time after Cyanide Injection

Normal mice in the control group (n = 8) died 2.25 ± 0.31 min after injection of potassium cyanide. However, the animals of the experimental group (n = 8) exposed to 4 runs survived for 9.38 ± 2.43 min after the injection, 4.1 times as long as the controls ($p < 0.01$).

Mandibular Breathing in vitro

The pattern of residual jaw movement and mandibular respiration of the isolated head could be divided into 4 successive phases: apnea I (latency), breathing I with high frequency, apnea II, and breathing II with low frequency based on the jaw movement curve (fig. 3).

The duration of breathing in phase II and apnea in phase I and II is shown in figure 3 and table 2. In the hypoxia-tolerant group, these durations were significantly longer than in the control group, except for breathing in phase I.

The number of phase I breaths in the hypoxia-tolerant group was significantly smaller than that in the controls, whereas the number of breaths in phase II and the total number were similar in the two groups (table 3). The respiration rate of the isolated head in hypoxia-tolerant group was thus certainly lower than that of controls (table 3).

Survival Time of Medulla and Spinal Cord in vitro

The survival times of the isolated medulla and the isolated spinal cord of the hypoxia-tolerant group were, respectively, 124 and 66 s in average. These were 5 and 3 times those of the controls (fig. 3, 4). The prolongation of medulla survival in the resistant group was mainly due to the prolongation of the apnea (fig. 3, 4, table 2).

Antihypoxic Effect of Brain Homogenate

The survival time in the hypobaric chamber of the group injected with brain supernatant from hypoxia-resistant mice (C) was about double that of the saline control group (A), and the non-hypoxia-exposed controls (B) (table 4). Statistically, the value in group C was significantly greater than that in either group A or B, and no significant difference between group A and B was seen.

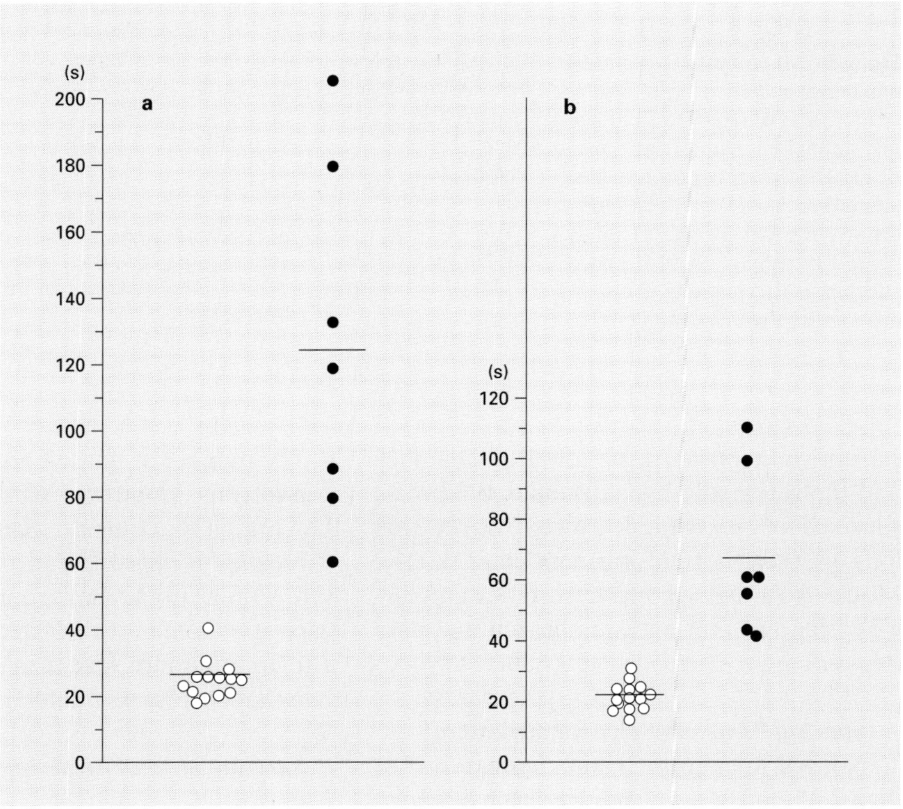

Fig. 4. Survival time of the medulla oblongate (**a**) and spinal cord (**b**) after decapitation. Open circles represent values taken from the control group preexposed to hypoxia, and closed circles represent the experimental group with repetitive exposure to hypoxia for 5 runs. The results indicate a kind of quickly developing adaptation with increased tolerance, and a very low but stable life action level achieved by acute and repetitive exposure to progressive autohypoxia.

Table 3. Number and rate ($\bar{x}$ ± SD) of mandibular breathing following decapitation

	Total	Phase I	Phase II
Mandibular breathing, n			
Control (C)	10.8 ± 0.42	5.9 ± 0.52	4.9 ± 0.42
Experimental (E)	8.7 ± 1.22	3.1 ± 0.58**	5.6 ± 1.38
E/C	0.8	0.5	1.1
Mandibular breathing rate			
Control (C)	0.44 ± 0.07	0.92 ± 0.31	0.32 ± 0.09
Experimental (E)	0.07 ± 0.03***	0.31 ± 0.17**	0.07 ± 0.05***
E/C	0.2	0.2	0.2

** $p < 0.01$ and *** $p < 0.001$, respectively, compared with the control group.

Table 4. Survival time (min, $\bar{x} \pm SD$) in hypobaric chamber

	Controls A	Non-hypoxia-exposed controls	Hypoxia resistant
n	15	15	15
Mean ± SE	13.20±4.8	11.60±3.5	24.30±6.2*
Ratio	1	0.88	1.83
		1	2.09

* $p < 0.05$, compared with group A and B.

Discussion

It is thought that there should be at least three factors – low oxygen, high CO_2, and low atmospheric pressure – involved in the airless condition in the present study. It is, however, generally recognized that the main consequence is hypoxia and the procedure is simply described as 'auto-hypoxia' [4]. This was confirmed in our preliminary study, when the CO_2 was absorbed by calcium hydroxide and the atmospheric pressure was kept constant with a capsule, leaving only hypoxia. The suggestion therefore arises that increased tolerance to hypoxia or adaptation to hypoxia is produced by hypoxia itself. This is verified by the long survival in the hypobaric chamber and the resistance to cyanide toxicity.

The adaptation seems to be characterized by at least four aspects: (1) adaptation to hypoxia develops quickly, in the order of minutes; (2) the tolerance increments in successive runs are much greater, being 2, 4, 6, 8 times as long in the 2nd, 3rd, 4th and 5th runs as in the 1st run, respectively, and the survival time in the hypoxia-exposed group was as long as 86 times that in the normal controls; (3) the disappearance of this adaptation is very rapid; it does not last to the next day or the 3rd day. Actually, there is no apparent increase in tolerance time if the interval between runs is prolonged to more than 15 min [unpubl. result], and (4) the level of life activity during the adaptation is low but stable, with less requirement for energy.

The above-mentioned characteristics are very different from the well-known chronic adaptation to hypoxia. It is, therefore reasonable to call this quickly formed and transient adaptation, 'acute adaptation', to distinguish it from the classical chronic adaptation. Such adaptation may also be classified as passive adaptation in view of the low life level compared to chronic adaptation which may thus be called active adaptation since it is characterized by fighting for more oxygen to expend energy.

Similar to what happened in vivo, as mentioned above, the isolated brain after repetitive exposure to hypoxia is characterized by long-lasting activity at a low level. The similarity suggests some correlation between isolated and intact brains.

It is generally recognized that respiration in phases I and II of the isolated head is determined, respectively, by aerobic and anaerobic metabolism in the respiratory center of the medulla oblongata [12–14]. The prominence of phase II of the isolated brain compared to phase I in the present study indicates that the long-lasting and low level of both activity and duration in both intact and isolated brains might be related to the anaerobic metabolism. When the energy supply to the mammalian brain is markedly decreased by anoxia, for a short time, energy requirements are curtailed by suppression of the nervous system, and energy supply is enhanced by increased cerebral blood flow and glycolysis [1].

Anoxia-tolerant species, like the turtle, apparently invoke the above mechanism to reduce energy expenditure, and are able to reduce their energy costs to a level that can be met by a greatly decreased oxygen supply from anaerobic glycolysis [1]. Inherent cellular properties in newborn [15] might also develop through repetitive exposure to hypoxia.

In addition, there should be other factors responsible for the maintenance of life activity at a low level. This is strongly suggested by observations in the present study that the hypoxia-resistant animals' brains contain some neurochemicals or metabolites that are extractable, transferable, and can permeate the blood-brain barrier to increase the receiver animal's tolerance to hypoxia. Further neurochemical study is needed to explore the nature of this kind of antihypoxia.

The options available to a living organism against change in environmental conditions range within two extremes: (a) regulatory mechanisms protect the internal conditions in an attempt to maintain constancy against environmental challenges, and (b) the internal state fluctuates to conform to external changes. The same ranges of options are available against hypoxia [16, 17]. At the one end, in chronic and active adaptation to hypoxia, the strategy for increasing tolerance to hypoxia rests on an increase in activity of many functioning systems, including the respiratory system, blood, circulation, and other organs and tissues, to keep higher levels of oxygen in arteries and cells. At the opposite end, all functional systems maintain low levels of ability and no advantage would be achieved even if these systems could increase their activity in acute and passive adaptation. Therefore, something must happen to the tissues and cells, especially in the brain, to increase tolerance to hypoxia while keeping low and stable levels of vital activity [2, 17, 18].

It was probably J.J.C. Le Gallois, in the 19th century, who first noted that newborn mammals are more resistant to anoxia than adults. This finding was later confirmed by other researchers and there is evidence that central neurons in newborn mammals survive longer than neurons in adults during oxygen deprivation [15, 18–20]. The greater resistance of younger mice in the present study seems to agree with the reports on newborn animals.

Scientists have been modeling ischemic stroke in animals for over 150 years and have devised many ingenious methods to try to mimic the human conditions. It is essential that physiologically controlled, reproducible in vivo animal models be used for systematic study of the pathophysiology and treatment of cerebral ischemia/hypoxia. Rigorous histopathologic, biochemical and physiological studies often require invasive surgical procedures, and direct access to brain tissue. Events occurring in the very early stages of ischemia should be thoroughly studied. Adaptive changes that developed acutely through the repetition of hypoxic exposure may serve as a model to help elucidate the physiological and biochemical basis of stroke, lung disorders, cardiac ischemia, and other nonclinical situations.

Acknowledgement

This project was supported by the National Natural Science Foundation of China (No. 39670271) and Beijing Natural Science Foundation (No. 7962009).

References

1 Lutz PL: Mechanisms for anoxic survival in the vertebrate brain. Annu Rev Physiol 1992;54:601–618.
2 Nesarajah MS, Matalon S, Krasneiy JA, et al: Cardiac output and regional oxygen transport in acutely hypoxic conscious sheep. Respir Physiol 1983;53:161–172.
3 Ginsberg MD, Busto R: Rodent models of cerebral ischemia. Stroke 1989;20:1627–1642.
4 Marshall JM, Metcalfe JD: Analysis of the cardiovascular changes induced in the rat by graded levels of systemic hypoxia. J Physiol (Lond) 1988;407:385–403.
5 Cartheuser CF: Progressive hypoxia until brain electrical silence: A useful model for studying protective interventions. Can J Physiol Pharmacol 1986;66:1398–1460.
6 Ryasina TV, Koshelev VB, Krushinsky AL, et al: The role of short-term hypobaric hypoxia in prevention of disorders of the cerebral circulation in rats during acustic stress. Brain Res 1988;473:153–156.
7 Schurr A: Adaptation of adult rat brain tissue to anoxia and hypoxia in vitro. Brain Res 1986;374:244–248.
8 Schurr A, Rigor BM: Cerebral ischemia revisited: New insights as revealed using in vitro brain slice preparation. Experientia 1989;45:684–694.
9 Walter K, Linas R: Electrophysiological activity recorded from the cerebral cortex of an isolated mammalian brain maintained in vitro. Soc Neurosci Abstr 1982;8:935.
10 Selle WA, Witten TA: Survival of the respiratory (gasping) mechanism in young animals subjected to anoxia. Proc Soc Biol Med 1941;47:495–497.
11 Jilek L, Mourek J, Trogan S: The influence of malonate on resistance to nitrogen anoxia and on the persistence of certain reflex during ontogeny of the rat. Physiol Bohemoslov 1961;10:267–275.
12 Hiestand WA, Tschirgi RD, Miller HR: The influence of glycolytic substances on survival of the primitive respiratory center in the ischemic rat head. Am J Physiol 1944;142:153–157.
13 Opitz E, Saathoff J: Überlebenszeit des primitiven Schnappatmungszentrums bei verschiedenen Warmblüter-Spezies vor und nach Höhenakklimatisation. Pflügers Arch Ges Physiol 1952;255:485–491.
14 Tschirgi RD, Gerard RW: The carotid-mandibular reflex in acute respiratory failure. Am J Physiol 1947;150:358–364.
15 Haddad GG, Donnelly DF: O_2 deprivation induces a major depolarization in brainstem neurons in the adult but not in the neonatal rat. J Physiol (Lond) 1990;429:411–428.
16 Lu GW: Adaptation to hypoxia via tissue and cell approaches; in Pan SC (ed): Advances in Pathophysiology. Beijing, People's Health Publishing. 1963, pp 196–237.
17 Mortola JP: Hypoxic hypometabolism in mammals. News Physiol Sci 1993;8:79–81.
18 Steinberg GK, Panahian N, Sun GH, et al: Interrupted, repeated arterial occlusion causes less cerebral ischemic damage than non-interrupted transient occlusion in a focal ischemic model. News Physiol Sci 1993;19:636.
19 Cherubini E, Ben-Ari Y, Krnjevic K: Anoxia produces smaller changes in synaptic transmission, membrane potential and input resistance in immature rat hippocampus. J Neurophysiol 1989;62:882–895.
20 Jiang C, Xia Y, Haddad GG: Role of ATP sensitive K+ channels during anoxia: Major differences between rat (newborn, adult) and turtle. J Physiol (Lond) 1992;448:599–612.

Biological Signals and Receptors

Biol Signals Recept 1999;8:256–260

Received: October 15, 1998
Accepted: October 30, 1998

Changes of Superoxide Dismutase, Glutathione Perioxidase and Lipid Peroxides in the Brain of Mice Preconditioned by Hypoxia

Chun-Li Duan[a] Fu-Sheng Yan[b] Xue-Ying Song[b] Guo-Wei Lu[c]

[a]Beijing Institute of Neurosciences and Departments of [b]Chemistry, and [c]Neurobiology, Capital University of Medical Sciences, Beijing, China

Key Words
Hypoxic preconditioning · Superoxide dismutase · Glutathione peroxidase · Lipid peroxides · Mouse

Abstract
We have developed an animal model of hypoxic preconditioning and assumed that oxygen radicals and their endogenous scavenging enzymes may play an important role in the preconditioning. To test this hypothesis, activities of superoxide dismutase (SOD), glutathione peroxidase (GSH-Px) and the content of lipid peroxides (LPO) were measured during the preconditioning. Compared with unpreconditioned control animals, in animals exposed to hypoxia only once, the activities of SOD and GSH-Px in whole brain were found to be significantly decreased while the LPO content in the hippocampus significantly increased. However, those in animals exposed to 4 runs of hypoxia tended to return to control levels and were lower than those in animals exposed to 1 and 2 runs of hypoxia. Our results indicate that the oxygen radicals and their specific scavenging enzymes seem to be involved in the development of tolerance to hypoxia.

Introduction

Ischemia-hypoxia is a common clinical physiopathological phenomenon. It is well known that under some pathological conditions, oxygen radicals are injurious to organs [1–3], so-called oxygen toxicity. There are many reports about the action of oxygen radicals in the injury of depriving oxygen-reoxygen (including ischemia-reperfusion) [4, 5], and some advances in developing oxygen radical scavengers have been made [6]. How-

KARGER
Fax + 41 61 306 12 34
E-Mail karger@karger.ch
www.karger.com

1422–4933/99/0085–0256$17.50/0

Accessible online at:
http://BioMedNet.com/karger

Chun-Li Duan
Beijing Institute of Neurosciences
Capital University of Medical Sciences
Beijing 100054 (China)

ever, to date little is known regarding the relationship between oxygen radicals and acute hypoxic preconditioning. The present study assessed changes in cerebral oxygen radicals and their endogenous scavengers superoxide dismutase (SOD) and glutathione peroxidase (GSH-Px) in relation to the development of acute hypoxic tolerance in our well-developed model of hypoxic preconditioning [7–9].

Materials and Methods

Animal Model

Adult and healthy male and female BALB/c and Kunming mice (16–20 g) were provided by the animal department of our university. The mice were randomly grouped by 4 to reproduce the model [7]. Briefly, the mouse was placed in a jar containing fresh air and made airtight with a rubber stopper. The animal was immediately removed and transferred to another jar containing fresh air as soon as gasping appeared. The transfer was repeated for 4 or 5 runs. The original time when gasping appeared in each run was normalized to standard tolerance time [8].

Apparatus and Reagents

UV-2201, UV/VIS spectrophotometer, RF-5000 fluorescence spectrophotometer (SHIMMADZU, Japan) and table-type high-speed freezing centrifuge (Beckman, USA) were used. SOD and reduced glutathione (GSH) were purchased from Boehringer Mannheim, Germany; 5.5′-Dithiobis-(2-nitrobenzonic acid) (DTNB), 1,1,3,3-tetraethoxypropane and sodium azide were from Sigma, USA. The remaining reagents were of domestic biochemical or analytical grade.

Preparation of Homogenate and Assays Used

Following exposure of mice to 1, 2 or 4 runs of hypoxia, the mice were rapidly decapitated. Their whole brains and hippocampuses were removed on ice-cold plates. The tissues were rinsed by ice-cold physiological saline and sucked up by filter paper. After precise weighing, the whole brains were homogenized in PBS (pH 7.8, containing 0.1 mmol/l EDTA) for 20% (w/v) homogenates at 0 °C. The homogenates were frozen and thawed three times, and centrifuged at 24,000 *g* at 0–4 °C for 30 min. After centrifugation, the supernatants were assayed for SOD activity according to a modified pyrogallol antioxidation method [9]. The activity of GSH-Px was determined by the DTNB direct method [10]. The hippocampal tissues were homogenized in physiological saline at 0 °C, and the homogenates (1%) were centrifuged for 10 min at 3,000 *g* at 0–4 °C. The supernatants were assayed for lipid peroxide (LPO) content by thiobarbituric acid fluorophotometry [11] (since we had tested the LPO content in the whole brain previously, we tested the LPO content in the hippocampus in order to make a comparison between them). The SOD activity was expressed in U/mg protein, and 1 U was defined as the amount of enzyme that inhibits the auto-oxidation rate per milliliter reaction solution by 50% under conditions of 25 °C, pH 8.2 and deducting the nonenzyme reaction. The GSH-Px activity was expressed as GSH concentration reduction per milligram protein and per minute (μmol/l·min·mg protein) and deducting the nonenzyme reaction. The LPO content was expressed per gram wet tissue containing malone dialdehyde (nmol/g). The protein level was assayed by the method of Lowry et al. [12].

Data Processing and Statistics

The values were expressed as mean ± SD and subjected to analysis of variance using the SYSTAT software and a t test for matched pairs. The level of significance was $p < 0.05$.

Results

Tolerance Time to Hypoxia

The standard tolerance times of mice to hypoxia in different runs are listed in table 1.

As shown in table 1, the tolerance time of mice to hypoxia progressively increased with acute and repeated exposure of hypoxia. This regular increase was consistent with previously published results [7, 13–16].

SOD Activity

SOD activities in the brains of mice exposed to different runs of hypoxia are shown in table 2. The activities of SOD in the mice exposed to hypoxia were significantly higher than those in the control group. However, following exposure to 4 runs of hypoxia, the activities of SOD were significantly lower than

Table 1. Standard tolerance time (Tt)[1] of mice exposed to hypoxia for different runs (min, mean ± SD, n = 20)

	Run 1	Run 2	Run 3	Run 4
Tt	17.20±5.23	31.85±4.34***	57.75±7.30***	106.25±6.07***
Ratio	1.00	1.85	3.36	6.18

*** $p < 0.01$ vs. run 1.

[1] $$T = \frac{T_0}{V_e} \times 100 = \frac{t_1 - t_0}{V_0 - V_a} \times 100 = \frac{t_1 - t_0}{V_0 - W_a/d_a} \times 100 = \frac{t_1 - t_0}{V_0 - W_a/0.94} \times 100,$$

where T: standard tolerance time (min), T_0: original tolerance time (min), $t_1 - t_0$: the time from beginning airtight to appearing gasping breath (min), V_e: the effective air volume (ml), V_0: the volume of the jar (ml), V_a: the volume of the mouse (ml), W_a: the weight of the mouse (g), d_a: the density of the mouse (g/ml). Its values are between 0.92 and 1.00 as concluded from many tests, and its mean value is 0.94.

Table 2. Activities of SOD in the brains of mice exposed to hypoxia for different runs (IU/mg Pro, mean ± SD, n = 10)

	Run 0	Run 1	Run 2	Run 4
SOD	23.48±1.09	30.88±1.35***	34.07±1.02***	29.75±0.79***, ooo
Ratio	1.00	1.32	1.45	1.27

*** $p < 0.001$, vs. control; ooo $p < 0.001$, vs. run 2.

those in animals exposed to 2 runs of hypoxia and tended to return to control levels.

GSH-Px Activity

GSH-Px activities in the brains of mice exposed to different runs of hypoxia are shown in table 3. Table 3 shows that the activities of GSH-Px in the mice exposed to hypoxia were significantly lower than those in the control group. However, in the animal exposed to 4 runs of hypoxia, the activities of GSH-Px in their brains were significantly higher than those in the group exposed to 2 runs of hypoxia and tended to close to the level in the control group.

LPO Content

LPO contents in the hippocampus of mice exposed to different runs of hypoxia are listed in table 4. As seen in table 4, the contents of LPO in groups exposed to hypoxia were significantly higher than those in the control group. However, when the animals were exposed to 4 runs of hypoxia, the contents of their cerebral LPO were significantly lower than those in the group exposed to 2 runs of hypoxia, and a decreasing tendency was shown. This tendency in the hippocampus is consistent with that in whole brain [13].

Table 3. Activities of GSH-Px in the brains of mice exposed to hypoxia for different runs (μmol/l·min·Pro, mean ± SD, n = 13)

	Run 0	Run 1	Run 2	Run 4
GSH-Px	12.33 ± 1.54	8.42 ± 0.93***	4.22 ± 1.71***	9.06 ± 1.67***,°°°
Ratio	1.00	0.68	0.34	0.73

*** $p < 0.001$, vs. control; °°° $p < 0.001$, run 4 vs. run 2.

Table 4. Contents of LPO in the hippocampus of mice exposed to hypoxia for different runs (nmol/g, mean ± SD, n = 10)

	Run 0	Run 1	Run 2	Run 4
LPO	283 ± 57	614 ± 33***	984 ± 85***	330 ± 62***,°°°
Ratio	1.00	2.17	3.48	1.17

*** $p < 0.001$, vs. control; °°° $p < 0.001$, vs. run 2.

Discussion

The brain is rich in polyunsaturated fatty acids, has a higher iron content, is poor in catalase activity and has only moderate activities of SOD and GSH-Px. The brain may, therefore, be especially prone to radical damage, initiating lipid peroxidation reactions and producing large quantities of LPO. SOD and GSH-Px are important endogenous enzymes for scavenging free radicals, eventually converting free radicals to water. The content of LPO represents the extent of free-radical damage to the organ and indirectly reflects the quantity of free radicals. The results of this study show that after exposure to hypoxia, SOD activity in mouse brain and LPO content in mouse hippocampus were significantly increased and GSH-Px activity in mouse brain was significantly decreased. However, after exposure to 4 runs of hypoxia, they all tended to return to control levels. These tendencies may be due to the following reasons. At the initial phase of hypoxia, energy metabolism is disturbed. This leads ATP to degrade and produce more xanthine and hypoxanthine. It also induces increases in cytosolic free Ca^{2+} and causes xanthine dehydrogenase to convert to xanthine oxidase. The latter oxidizes xanthine to hypoxanthine and then to uric acid, simultaneously reducing of O_2 to both $O^{2\bullet-}$ and H_2O_2. In addition, the increased cytosolic free Ca^{2+} leads to rapid hydrolysis of phospholipids and releases free arachidonic acid, which can produce $O^{2\bullet-}$ in its metabolic process. The increased $O^{2\bullet-}$ may augment SOD activity. Alternatively it may inhibit GSH-Px activity. The LPO content is then increased. Following increasing hypoxic exposure runs, the mice may develop some adaptive mechanisms: they may regulate their temperature and decrease their energy requirement and consumption; their ATP and ATPase activity levels may thus be maintained and the damaged ionic homeostasis, especially Ca^{2+}, may be corrected: for the above reasons, the product increase in $O^{2\bullet-}$ stops; in addition to higher SOD activity, GSH-Px activity rises again. The ability of scavenging $O^{2\bullet-}$ is thus enhanced and LPO content is lowered. This explanation seems to be consistent with our previous results [14–16]. The results in the present study also indicate that an increase in SOD activity is unable to mitigate or stop the injury caused by the oxygen radicals. However, when the increase in SOD activity is combined with other related enzymes, such as GSH-Px, CATase, oxygen radicals can be effectively scavenged. The above findings have to be considered when the antioxidant is used to cure diseases involving oxygen stress.

Acknowledgment

This work was supported by the National Natural Science Foundation of China (Nc. 39670271) and Natural Science Foundation of Beijing (No. 7962009).

References

1 Halliwell B: Reactive oxygen species and the central nervous system. J Neurochem 1992;59:1609–1622.
2 Taniguchi N: Clinical significances of superoxide dismutase: Changes in aging, diabetes, ischemia and cancer. Adv Clin Chem 1992;29:17–23.
3 Halliwell B: Free radicals, antioxidants and human disease: Curiosity, cause, or consequence? Lancet 1994; 334:721–724.
4 Traystman RJ, Kirsch JR, Koehler RC: Oxygen radical mechanisms of brain injury following ischemia and reperfusion. J Appl Physiol 1991;71: 1185–1195.
5 Siesjo BK: A new perspective on ischemic brain damage? Prog Brain Res 1993;96:1–9.
6 Choi DW: Cerebral hypoxia: Some new approaches and unanswered questions. J Neurosci 1990;10: 2493–2501.
7 Lu GW, Shi MT, Li L, An YY: Effects of repeated exposure to hypoxia on hypoxia tolerance in mice (in Chinese). Chin J Pathophysiol 1992;8:426–429.
8 Lu GW, Ding DW, Shi MT: Acute adaptation of mice to hypoxic hypoxia. Biol Signals Recept 1999;8: 247–255.
9 Deng BY, Yuan QS, Li WJ: Superoxide dismutase assayed by a modified pyrogallol antioxidant method (in Chinese). Progr Biochem Biophys 1991;18:163.
10 Xia YM, Zhu LZ: The determination of glutathione peroxidase in blood and tissue – DTNB direct method (in Chinese). J Hyg Res 1987;16:29–33.
11 Tanizawa H, Sazuka Y: Micro-determination of lipoperoxide in the mouse myocardium by thiobarbituric acid fluorophotometry. Chem Pharm Bull (Tokyo) 1981;29:2910–2914.
12 Lowry OH, Rosebrough NJ, Farr AL, Randall RJ: Protein measurement with the Folin phenol reagent. J Biol Chem 1951;193:265–275.
13 Xu RX, Zhou YL, Lu GW: Effects of acute repetitive hypoxia on lipid peroxide levels in mouse brain (in Chinese). Basic Med Sci Clin 1994; 14:464–466.
14 Zhang JN, Yan SL, Liu YL: Changes of Na^+-K^+-ATPase and Ca^{2+}-ATPase activities in brain of mice exposed to hypoxia (in Chinese). Chin J Appl Phys 1994;10:237.
15 Liu HM, Zhu DS, Li HJ: The influence of acute repetitive hypoxia on free fatty acids in the mouse brain (in Chinese). Basic Med Sci Clin 1993;13:382–384.
16 Yan FS, Song XY, Liu JH, Lu GW: Changes of phospholipid composition in mouse brain acutely exposed to hypoxia (in Chinese). Chin J Pathophysiol 1995;11:375–377.

Biological Signals and Receptors

Biol Signals Recept 1999;8:261–266

Received: November 13, 1998
Accepted: February 12, 1999

Changes in Phospholipids and Free Fatty Acids in the Brains of Mice Preconditioned by Hypoxia

Chun-Li Duan[d] Fu-Sheng Yan[a] Guo-Wei Lu[b]
Hui-Min Liu[c] Na Yin[a]

[a]Departments of Hygienic-Chemistry, [b]Neurobiology and [c]Chemistry, and
[d]Beijing Institute of Neurosciences, Capital University of Medical Sciences, Beijing, China

Key Words

Hypoxic preconditioning · Phospholipids · Free fatty acids

Abstract

Changes in the composition and contents of phospholipids and free fatty acids were observed and compared in three groups: (A) unpreconditoned normal controls, (B) exposure to 1 run of hypoxia and (C) exposure to 4 runs of hypoxia. In group B, the content of phosphatidyl ethanolamine (PE), phosphatidyl serine (PS) and free fatty acids (FFAs) increased significantly and the content of phosphatidyl choline (PC) and sphingomyelin (SM) decreased significantly. While in group C the content of PE, PS, PC and FFAs changed significantly when compared with that of group B, all phospholipid (except SM) and FFA contents tended to decrease to the level of group A. No new FFA was seen in the brain homogenates in any of the three groups. These results suggest that the changes in the content of mouse brain phospholipids and FFAs may be adaptive and involved in the animals' tolerance to hypoxia.

Introduction

The study of hypoxic-ischemic preconditioning is now increasing. Ischemia induces the breakdown of membrane phospholipids and the accumulation of free fatty acids (FFAs), including arachidonic acid. This release of fatty acids caused by ischemia was first described by Bazan [1] in 1970 and is thus called the Bazan effect. Since then, a large number of reports on lipid peroxidation

KARGER

Fax + 41 61 306 12 34
E-Mail karger@karger.ch
www.karger.com

1422–4933/99/0085–0261$17.50/0

Accessible online at:
http://BioMedNet.com/karger

Chun-Li Duan
Beijing Institute of Neurosciences
Capital University of Medical Sciences
Beijing 100054 (China)

of polyunsaturated fatty acids during and after hypoxia have been published [2, 3]. However, there are few reports on the changes in the composition and content of phospholipids and free fatty acids (FFAs) in acute hypoxic preconditioning. The present study is aimed at exploring the changes in composition and content of phospholipids and FFAs in the brains of animals repeatedly exposed to hypoxia. Our studies may provide important insights into the mechanism of acute hypoxic preconditioning.

Materials and Methods

Animal Model

Healthy adult male and female BALB/c and Kunming mice (17.0–22.0 g) were provided by the animal department of our university. The mice were divided randomly into three groups: (A) unpreconditioned normal control group, (B) those exposed to 1 run of hypoxia and (C) those exposed to 4 runs of hypoxia. The detailed procedure for producing the model of hypoxic preconditioning was elaborately described previously [4]. Briefly, the mouse was placed in a jar containing fresh air and the jar was made airtight with a rubber stopper. The animal was removed immediately and transferred into another similar jar containing fresh air when it started gasping. The transfer was repeated for 4 runs. The animal's original time of gasping appearance in each run was normalized to standard tolerance time [4].

Reagents

Palmitic acid methyl ester (16:0), palmitoleic acid methyl ester (16:1), stearic acid methyl ester (18:0), oleic acid methyl ester (18:1), linoleic acid methyl ester (18:2), linolenic acid methyl ester (18:3), arachidonic acid methyl ester (20:4) and nervonic acid methyl ester (24:1) were purchased from Sigma. n-Heptadecamoic acid (17:0) was from Merck. The remaining reagents were of domestic analytical grade.

Processes and Assays of the Samples

The mice exposed to different runs of hypoxia and controls were rapidly decapitated in the freezing condition. The whole brains were rinsed by ice-cold physiological saline and sucked up by filter paper and weighed.

Phospholipid Assay

The extract solutions were prepared, evaporated, condensed, and finally adjusted to 1.0 ml. Quantitative lipid solutions were applied onto a silica gel plate (5 × 10 cm) and developed by $CHCl_3$:CH_3OH:HAC:H_2O (5:4:1:0.2). Spots were detected by iodine vapor and were scraped off from the plate. The scraped silica gel powder was washed, collected, dried and then nitrated with HNO_3:H_2O_2 (2:1). After nitration, phosphorus reagent was added. The inorganic phosphorus was detected using a WFJ 80-1 spectrophotometer. The phospholipid concentrations were calculated.

FFA Assay

The homogenates were prepared with $CHCl_3$:CH_3OH (2:1, v/v) and methylated with BF_3-$(C_2H_5)_2O$-CH_3OH. For purification, liquid-liquid partition was used. The purified solution was condensed and dissolved in n-hexane. The FFAs were detected by gas chromatography according to the method of Huizhu-Xu et al. [5], modified as follows: SQ-206 gas chromatography; FID detector; 2 m × 3 mm stainless steel column; 10% DEGS/Chromosorb WAW DMCS 80–100 mesh; the initial temperature was 160°C, after 5 min, the temperature was raised to 170°C at the rate of 1°C/min, and finally to 195°C at the rate of 5°C/min; the temperature of the gasifying and detection chamber was 250°C; the carrier gases were nitrogen (0.4 kg/cm^2), hydrogen (0.4 kg/cm^2), air (0.6 kg/cm^2).

Statistical Analysis

Data were expressed as means ± SD. Statistical significance was determined by ANOVA analysis (F value) followed by a pair-matched t test. $p < 0.05$ was considered as statistically significant.

Results

Changes in Tolerance to Hypoxia

The standard tolerance time of mice to hypoxia in different runs is listed in table 1. As shown in the table, the tolerance time was progressively prolonged when the animals were acutely and repeatedly exposed to hypoxia. Its regular increase was consistent with previously published results [4].

Table 1. Standard tolerance time (T_t) of mice exposed to different runs of hypoxia (min, mean ± SD, n = 20)

	Run 1	Run 2	Run 3	Run 4
T_t	8.8±2.6	38.4±1.8***	58.4±3.3***	67.0±3.3***
Ratio	1.00	4.36	6.64	7.61

*** $p<0.001$ vs. run 1.

Table 2. Absorption values of cerebral phospholipids in different groups (mean ± SD, n = 20)

	PE	PS	PC	SM
Unpreconditioned control (A)	141.2±20.0	54.3±10.5	239.5±20.6	59.4±8.2
Exposure to 1 run of hypoxia (B)	351.4±32.2°	131.5±18.0°	123.7±15.0°	37.4±8.2°
Exposure to 4 runs of hypoxia (C)	205.1±27.6*	98.2±14.1*	158.5±18.7*	18.7±3.5*

° $p<0.001$ vs. A; * $p<0.001$ vs. B.

Changes in Cerebral Phospholipid Content

Each brain sample was separated by thin layer chromatography, and four phospholipid compositions were measured: phosphatidyl ethanolamine (PE), phosphatidyl serine (PS), phosphatidyl choline (PC) and sphingomyelin (SM). The phospholipid composition was detected separately. As shown in table 2 and figure 1, the PE and PS contents in the group exposed to 1 run of hypoxia were significantly higher than the mean content of the control group while the mean value in the group exposed to 4 runs of hypoxia was significantly lower than in the mice exposed to 1 run of hypoxia. The content of PC in the group exposed to 1 run of hypoxia was significantly lower than the mean of the control group and the PC content for mice exposed to hypoxia for 4 runs was lower than that for the control group, but higher than that for mice exposed to 1 run of hypoxia. The content of SM in mice exposed to 1 run of hypoxia was significantly lower than that of the control group while the SM content in mice exposed to 4 runs of hypoxia continued to decrease.

Changes in Contents of FFAs

As shown in table 3, the contents of palmitic acid (16:0), stearic acid (18:0), oleic acid (18:1) and arachidonic acid (20:4) were higher for the groups exposed to hypoxia than those for control mice. The results were similar to those of Lunt and Rowe [6]. The contents of the seven FFAs in mice exposed to 1 run of hypoxia were significantly higher than those for the control group (18:0, 18:2, 20:4, $p < 0.05$; 18:1, 18:3, 24:1, $p < 0.01$; 16:0, $p < 0.001$). No significant difference was seen in the contents of the eight FFAs between the group exposed to 4 runs of hypoxia and normal controls. Under the same gas chromatographic conditions, FFAs in the homogenates of different groups were not significantly different and no new FFA composition was found in the present study.

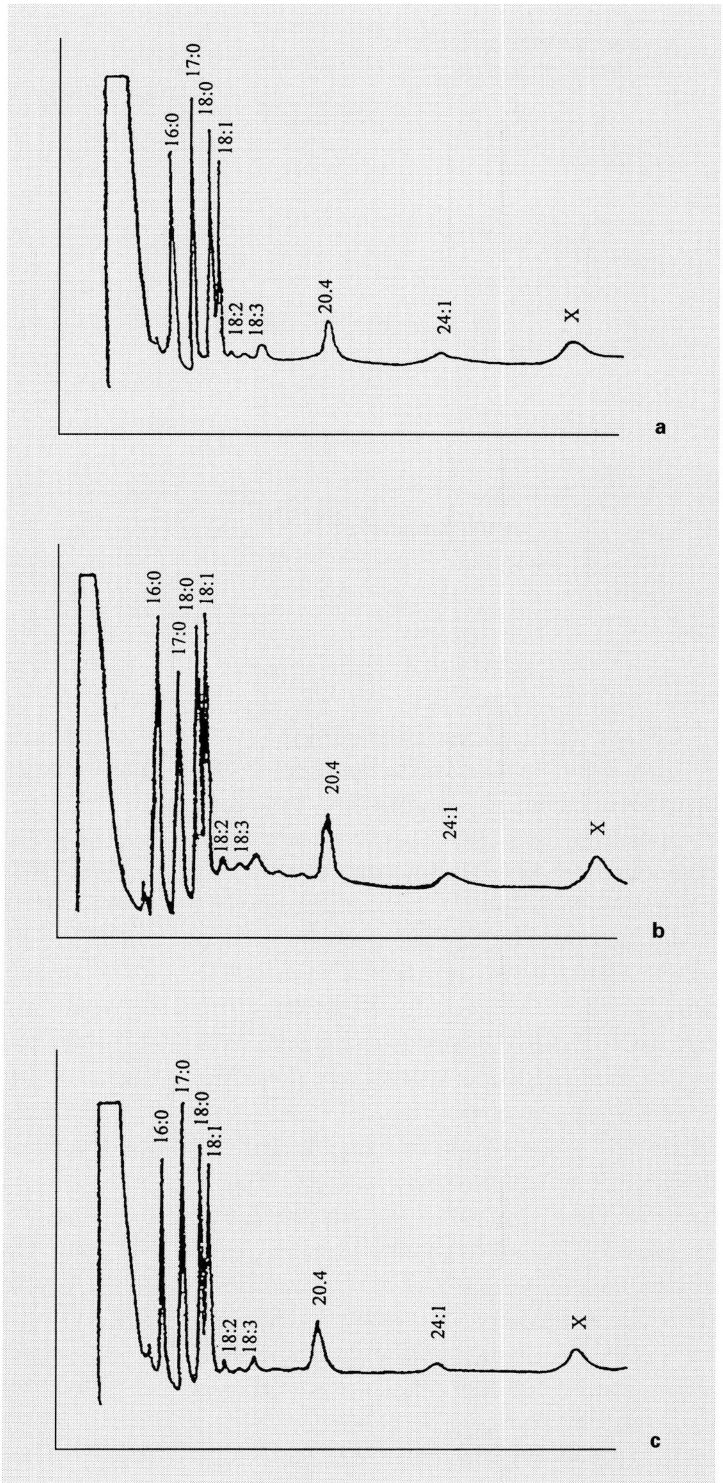

Fig. 1. Chromatograms of FFAs from mouse brain homogenates. **a** Controls. **b** Exposure to 1 run of hypoxia. **c** Exposure to 4 runs of hypoxia.

Table 3. Contents of FFAs in the mouse brains of different groups (mean ± SD, n = 9)

	16:0	16:1	18:0	18:1	18:2	18:3	20:4	24:1
Unpreconditioned control (A)	3.86±0.51	trace	2.59±0.13	3.25±0.28	0.33±0.01	0.42±0.14	1.72±0.28	0.48±0.17
Exposure to 1 run of hypoxia (B)	6.07±0.29***	trace	3.79±0.25*	4.70±0.55**	0.41±0.12*	0.65±0.16**	2.54±0.38*	0.68±0.12**
Exposure to 4 runs of hypoxia (C)	3.91±0.50	trace	2.63±0.26	3.06±0.26	0.32±0.01	0.52±0.17	1.67±0.28	0.55±0.13

* $p < 0.05$, ** $p < 0.01$, *** $p < 0.001$ vs. control.

Discussion

Lipids constitute about one half of brain tissue dry weight and phospholipids are the main components of the cytoplasmic neuronal membranes. These are made up of glycerol and polyunsaturated fatty acid chains and constitute an important factor in determining membrane fluidity. The breakdown of membrane phospholipids disrupts membrane ionic gradients and may be involved in the membrane damage caused by hypoxia. The present study indicates that after a single exposure to hypoxia, the contents of PE, PS and of seven FFAs in the brain tissue of mice increased significantly while the contents of PC and SM decreased significantly. After 4 runs of hypoxia, PE, PS, PC and FFAs showed a tendency to return to normal levels except for SM which continued to decrease, a tendency similar to the changes in Na^+-K^+-ATPase and Ca^{2+}-ATPase activities reported previously [7].

When the mice were initially exposed to hypoxia, the energy metabolism was disrupted and the activities of Na^+-K^+-ATPase and Ca^{2+}-ATPase were inhibited. These induce ionic homeostasis disturbance, especially calcium influx into the neuron results in stimulation of phospholipase C (Ca^{2+}-dependent) and phospholipase A (cAMP-dependent) [8, 9]. These enzymes are the well-known enzymes responsible for membrane lipid breakdown. In addition, a disturbance in energy metabolism leads to ATP degradation and increased cytosolic calcium activates xanthine oxidase. These actions may lead to the formation of oxygen free radicals, which may attack polyunsaturated fatty acids in the cell membrane and may induce phospholipid degradation and FFA formation. So with the initial phase of hypoxia, the contents of PC and SM decreased and the contents of FFAs, PE and PS increased, while after 4 exposures to hypoxia, the contents of PC, PE, PS and FFAs approached normal levels. Our results indicate that under hypoxic preconditioning, the animals may be developing a degree of adaptation to hypoxia. This may be due to the fact that mice regulate their body temperature and decrease their energy requirement and consumption. Their ATP and ATPase activity may thus be maintained and the damaged ionic homeostasis, especially $[Ca^{2+}]_i$, may be corrected. Further studies are needed to determine the mechanism and significance of the continuing decrease in SM content.

Acknowledgment

This work was supported by the National Natural Science Foundation of China (No. 39670271) and the Natural Science Foundation of Beijing (No. 7962009).

References

1 Bazan N: Effect of ischemia and electroconvulsive shock on free fatty acid pool in the brain. Biochim Biophys Acta 1970;218:1–16.

2 Traystaman RJ, Kirsch JR, Koehler RC: Oxygen radical mechanisms of brain injury following ischemia and reperfusion. J Appl Physiol 1991;71:1185–1195.

3 Yamamoto S: Enzymatic lipid peroxidation: Reactions of mammalian lipoxygenases. Free Radic Biol Med 1991;10:149–168.

4 Lu GW, Ding DW, Shi MT: Acute adaptation of mice to hypoxic hypoxia. Biol Signals Recept 1999;8:247–255.

5 Xu HZ, Chen RG, Zhang WL: Analysis of free fatty acid in human blood by gas chromatography (in Chinese). Acta Nutrimenta Sin 1986;8:165–169.

6 Lunt GG, Rowe CE: The production of unesterified fatty acid in brain. Biochim Biophys Acta 1968;152:681–693.

7 Zhang JN, Yan SL, Liu YL: Changes in Na^+-K^+-ATPase and Ca^{2+}-ATPase activities in brain of mice exposed to hypoxia (in Chinese). Chin J Appl Phys 1994;10:237.

8 Chien KR, Pfau RG, Farber JL: Ischemia myocardial injury: Prevention by chlorpromazine of an accelerated phospholipid and associated membrane dysfunction. Am J Pathol 1979;97:505–530.

9 Demerle-Pallaroly C, Lonchampt MO, Chabrier PE, Braquet P: Absence of implication of *L*-arginine/nitric oxide pathway on neuronal cell injury induced by *L*-glutamate or hypoxia. Biochem Biophys Res Commun 1991;181:456–464.

Biological Signals and Receptors

Biol Signals Recept 1999;8:267–274

Received: October 15, 1998
Accepted: October 30, 1998

Role of Excitatory Amino Acids in Hypoxic Preconditioning

Jinghui Xie[a] Guo-Wei Lu[b] Yan-Zhi Hou[b]

[a]Graduate College, University of Iowa, Iowa City, Iowa, USA, and
[b]Department of Neurobiology, Capital University of Medical Science, Beijing, China

Key Words

Excitatory amino acids · Hypoxic preconditioning · Ionotropic NMDA receptor · Aspartate · Ketamine

Abstract

We examined the effects of the extrinsic ionotropic NMDA receptor agonist (aspartate) and antagonist (ketamine) on the hypoxic preconditioning of mice and the concentration changes of intrinsic excitatory amino acids (EAAs), aspartate and glutamate, in the whole brain and different brain regions during preconditioning by an HPLC method. Our results showed that aspartate and ketamine significantly prolonged and shortened the standard tolerance time of mice during preconditioning and survival time in hypobaric chambers, respectively. After the 1st exposure, EAA concentrations in the whole brain and brain regions were increased. After run 4, they were decreased or maintained. It is suggested that the activation and suppression of ionotropic NMDA receptors is harmful and beneficial to hypoxic preconditioning, respectively. Degradation and/or inactivation of EAAs might be beneficial to the tolerance of mice to hypoxia.

Introduction

Hypoxia is a major pathophysiological process in cardiovascular and/or cerebral vascular diseases, as well as in other diseases, such as heart failure. It is also an important etiological factor in neuronal damage. During hypoxia, the concentrations of excitatory amino acids (EAAs) in the brain have been reported to be increased [1–5], their receptors activated, excitotoxicity induced and intracellular calcium overloaded, thus leading to hyp-

KARGER

Fax + 41 61 306 12 34
E-Mail karger@karger.ch
www.karger.com

1422–4933/99/0085–0267$17.50/0

Accessible online at:
http://BioMedNet.com/karger

Jinghui Xie
The University of Iowa, Graduate College
Neuroscience Program, 1119 Medical Laboratories
Iowa City, IA 52242 (USA)
E-Mail jhxie@public.east.cn.net

oxic brain damage [6, 7]. On the other hand, acute and repeated exposure to hypoxia can significantly enhance the tolerance of mice to hypoxia by preconditioning [8]. Further understanding of hypoxic preconditioning would help find better ways to protect neurons from hypoxic damage. The purpose of the present study was to observe the effects of the extrinsic ionotropic NMDA receptor agonist, aspartate, and antagonist, ketamine, on hypoxic preconditioning of mice, measure the concentration changes of intrinsic EAAs (aspartate and glutamate) in the whole brain and different brain regions (telecephalon, hippocampus, midbrain, pons cerebelli, medulla oblongata and cerebellum) during hypoxic preconditioning, and thus to explore their role in preconditioning.

Materials and Methods

Tolerance Time Measurements

Sixty-five Kunming mice of both sexes weighing 17–21 g were randomly divided into three groups: the asparatate (ASP), the normal saline (NS) and the ketamine (KET) group, with the NS group as control. 3 g/kg of aspartate, 3 ml/kg of normal saline and 100 mg/kg of ketamine were administered intraperitoneally, respectively. The laboratory temperature was in the range of 18–22 °C. Then the standard hypoxic tolerance time in each hypoxic run during preconditioning was examined.

Ten minutes after administration, the mice underwent 4 runs of acute repeated exposure to hypoxia, as indicated in our mouse preconditioning model [8]. The mice were put into jars with fresh air, whose volumes had been measured to be about 150 ml. Then the jars were sealed hermetically. The original tolerance time (T_0) was measured, indicated by the time duration from the beginning of exposure (t_0) to the appearance of gasping (t_1). The standard tolerance time (T_s) was calculated as following:

$$T_s = T_0/V_e \times 100 = (t_1 - t_0)/(V_0 - W_a/0.94) \times 100,$$

where V_e is the calculated effective volume of the jar, V_0 is the measured original volume of the jar, W_a is the animal's weight, and 0.94 is the density of the mouse measured in preliminary experiments.

Table 1. Gradient elution partition chromatography

Time	A	B
0–9 min, %	90.8	9.2
9–11 min, %	0	100
11–15 min, %	90.8	9.2

A = 0.1 mol/l acetate buffer. B = Methanol.

Survival Time Measurements

Forty-two Kunming mice were divided into three groups as above, according to their weight and sex. Fifteen minutes after administration, the mice were put into hypobaric chambers (P_{O_2} = 4.1 kPa, 30 mm Hg), and their survival time was measured.

EAA Concentration Measurements

Fifty-one Kunming mice were divided into three groups according to sex and weight: normal, hypoxic run 1 and hypoxic run 4. The heads of the mice were kept in –10 °C liquid nitrogen right after hypoxic exposure. The next day, the tissues of the whole brain (n = 10) and of the different brain regions (telencephalon, hippocampus, midbrain, pons cerebelli, medulla oblongata and cerebellum, n = 21) were isolated and weighed. One and 0.5 ml of pure water were added to 400 mg of the whole brain and regional brain tissues, respectively. Samples were homogenized at <0 °C and centrifuged at 13,500 rpm for 45 min under –4 °C. After addition of 100 µl of 10% trichloroacetic acid to the supernatants, they were centrifuged at 13,500 rpm for 25 min under –4 °C. The supernatants were adjusted to pH 7–8 with 1 mol/l NaOH and filtered with a 40-µm filter.

Twenty-two kinds of standard amino acids, including aspartate and glutamate, were measured exactly and smelted in 0.1 mol/l acetate buffer to receive 5 mmol/l of standard solution, which was diluted to 1.0 mmol/l and 500, 100, 50, and 10 µmol/l of standard solution, respectively.

The standard and supernatant samples were analyzed by HPLC with the *o*-phthaldialdehyde (OPA) precolumn derivatization technique. A reverse-phase C_{18} column (Nova Pak 150 × 3.9 nm, 4 µm, Waters, USA) was used in the HPLC system (HP 1050 liquid chromatograph, Hewlett, USA). The mobile phase composed of 0.1 mol/l acetate buffer (pH 6.95) and

Table 2. Standard hypoxic tolerance time (min, $\bar{x} \pm SD$) of NS, ASP, and KET groups, respectively

Group	n	Run of hypoxia exposure			
		1	2	3	4
NS	23	15.4 ± 1.6	$33.9 \pm 5.5^{**}$	$56.6 \pm 7.8^{**}$	$76.5 \pm 13.3^{**}$
ASP	21	12.8 ± 2.1^{a}	$27.4 \pm 4.2^{**, a}$	$51.0 \pm 6.8^{**, a}$	$68.3 \pm 7.1^{**, a}$
KET	21	$23.0 \pm 6.7^{**, b}$	$44.9 \pm 10.0^{**, b}$	$73.2 \pm 8.7^{**, b}$	$88.9 \pm 12.5^{**, b}$

* $p < 0.05$, ** $p < 0.01$, compared with preceding run within its group. [a] $p < 0.05$, [b] $p < 0.01$, compared with NS group.

methanol was delivered at a flow rate of 0.8 ml/min by a high pressure pump (HP 1050Q, Hewlett). After derivative reaction with OPA, the samples (20 μl) were injected into the HPLC system by an autosampler and eluted gradiently by HPLC (table 1). The contents of glutamate and aspartate in the samples were detected by a fluorescence detector with Ex = 450 nm and Em = 350 nm.

Statistics

SYSTAT statistics software was used to process the data, the t test was used for the comparison of T_s among groups, the paired t test for T_s within groups and survival time, and ANOVA for the changes in concentrations of aspartate and glutamate.

Results

T_s Changes

During preconditioning, the behavior of the NS group was the same as indicated in our previous research [8]. In the 1st hypoxic run, mice showed growing cyanosis and short breath. After 8–10 min, mice began to be restless. Later, the righting reactions and spontaneous movements of the mice disappeared, and they showed spasm-like actions and gasped for breath. In the 2nd hypoxic run, the manifestations of the mice were similar to those in the 1st run, except for their fewer spontaneous movements as well as their decreasing and delayed restlessness. During the 3rd and 4th run, mice were quiet with little spontaneous movements and showed deep, slow and regular breathing without significant restlessness. The T_s of mice significantly increased according to the proceeding run (table 2).

The ASP group showed more spontaneous movements and restlessness than the NS group during the 1st and 2nd hypoxic run. In the 3rd and 4th run, their manifestations were similar to those of the NS group. The KET group as quiet with much fewer spontaneous movements than the NS group. Mice breathed deeply and slowly. The T_s of the ASP and KET groups also increased subsequent to the proceeding run, but in each run, the T_s of the ASP and KET groups was significantly shorter or longer than that of the NS group, respectively (table 2).

Survival Time Changes

In the hypobaric chamber, the ASP and NS group showed increasing restlessness and cyanosis immediately. The KET group was quieter and breathed deeper and slower than the ASP group. Survival times of the ASP, NS and KET groups ($\bar{x} \pm SD$) were 1.4 ± 0.2,

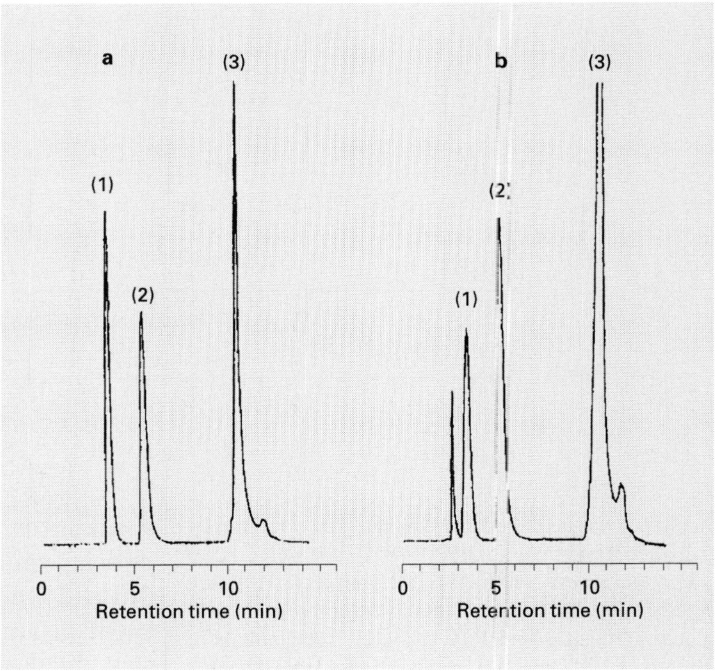

Fig. 1. HPLC chromatograms of an amino acid standard mixture (**a**) and the brain sample (**b**). Peaks: (1) = aspartate, (2) = glutamate, (3) = other amino acids.

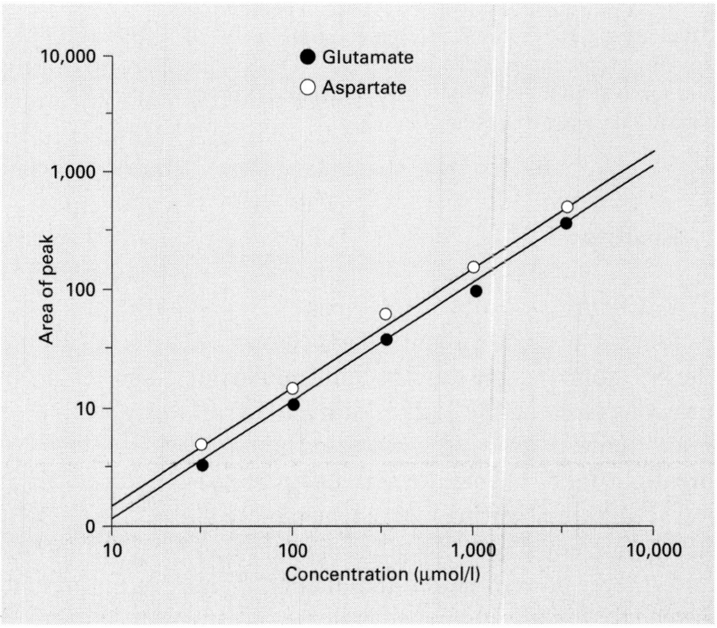

Fig. 2. Standard concentration curve of aspartate and glutamate. The X-axis represents the concentration of aspartate and glutamate. The Y-axis represents the peak are shown in chromatography.

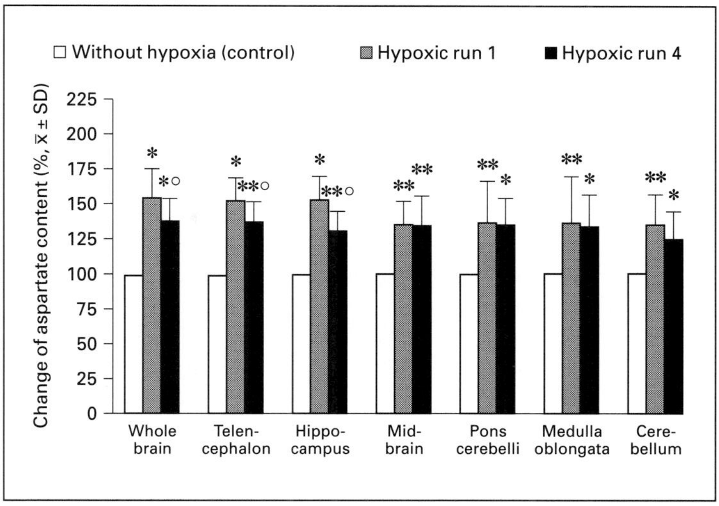

Fig. 3. Change (%, $\bar{x} \pm$ SD) of the aspartate content in the whole brain and different brain regions following hypoxic runs 1 and 4. The y-axis represents the percentage change when the value in the control group is regarded as 100%. The x-axis shows the whole brain (n = 30) and 4 different brain regions (n = 21 for each region). * $p < 0.05$, ** $p < 0.01$ compared with control (without hypoxia); ° $p < 0.05$ compared with hypoxic run 1.

1.6 ± 0.4, and 4.3 ± 0.7 min, respectively. Survival times of the ASP and KET group were significantly shorter ($p < 0.05$) or longer ($p < 0.01$) than that of the NS group, respectively.

Normal EAA Concentrations in the Brain and Their Changes

Normal Values of EAA Concentrations. The HPLC chromatograms of the standard amino acid solution and of a normal brain sample are shown in figure 1. The standard curve is shown in figure 2. Table 3 shows aspartate and glutamate concentrations in the group without exposure to hypoxia.

EAA Concentration Changes. After the first exposure, the aspartate and glutamate concentrations in the whole brain and the different brain regions were increased. After the 4th run, i.e. with the formation of preconditioning aspartate and glutamate concentrations in the whole brain, telencephalon and hippocampus were decreased, and that of glutamate in hippocampus had dropped to normal levels. In the midbrain, pons cerebelli and medulla oblongata, aspartate and glutamate concentrations were maintained at the same levels as those in the group of run 1. In the cerebellum, after preconditioning, the concentration of aspartate was kept at the same level as in the group of run 1, while that of glutamate dropped to normal (fig. 3, 4).

Table 3. Concentrations of aspartate and glutamate (μmol/g brain weight, $\bar{x} \pm$ SD) in the whole brain and different brain regions

Brain region	n	Aspartate	Glutamate
Whole brain	10	0.84±0.25	1.76±0.59
Telencephalon	7	0.83±0.32	1.76±0.66
Hippocampus	7	0.58±0.18	1.79±0.63
Midbrain	7	0.49±0.16	1.07±0.26
Pons cerebelli	7	0.56±0.21	1.53±0.59
Medulla oblongata	7	0.60±0.24	1.50±0.40
Cerebellum	7	0.80±0.26	1.69±0.49

Fig. 4. Change (%, $\bar{x} \pm SD$) of the glutamate content in the whole brain and different brain regions following hypoxic runs 1 and 4. The y-axis represents the percentage change when the value in the control group is regarded as 100%. The x-axis shows the whole brain (n = 30) and 4 different brain regions (n = 21 for each region). * $p < 0.05$, ** $p < 0.01$ compared with control (without hypoxia); ○ $p < 0.05$ compared with hypoxic run 1.

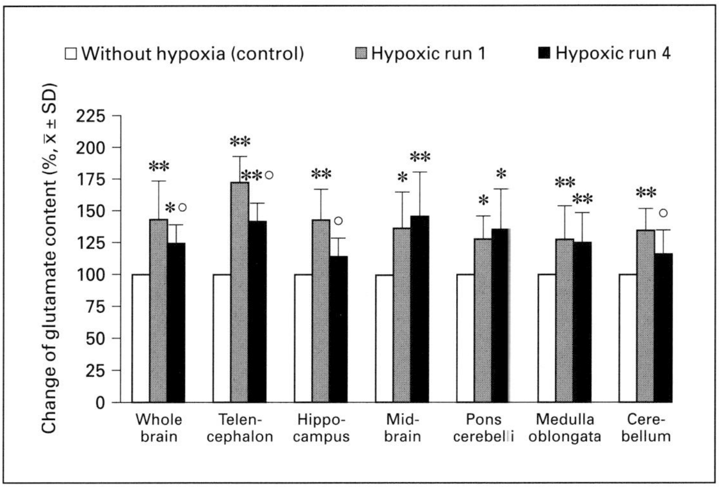

Discussion

The tolerance of the central nervous system is essential to survival when animals and humans are exposed to a hypoxic condition. EAAs and their receptors are thought to play an important role in hypoxic neuronal damage when extracellular EAAs are accumulated, their receptors activated, calcium is overloaded and neuronal death occurs, i.e. so-called EAA excitatoxicity [6, 7].

In the normal brain, the concentration of glutamate is 12–13 mmol/l, consisting mainly of intracellular glutamate. The extracellular glutamate maintains 1 µmol/l or so [9], but no higher than 10 µmol/l. It has been reported that the content of aspartate and glutamate is increased after hypoxia [1–5], which is also shown in the present study. In hypoxia, because of ATP exhaustion, EAAs are released without vesiculation, acting independently on calcium. Besides, the depolarization of neurons exacerbates EAA release. Furthermore, depolarization and accumulation of arachidonic acids inhibit the uptake of EAAs. As a result, free EAAs in the brain increase during hypoxia.

NMDA EAAs AMPA/KA, and metabotropic receptors participate in excitotoxicity [10–16]. It has been proved that the activation of NMDA receptors results in Ca^{2+} influx, and that of AMPA/KAs causes Na^+ influx, simultaneous Cl^- and H_2O influx, and neuron acute swelling. Meanwhile, the activation of metabotropic receptors activates coupled G-protein, and through the second messengers causes Ca^{2+} influx and overload [17]. Calcium overload is supposed to be the common way of neuronal death, in which free oxygen radicals [2, 18] and nitric oxide are also involved [19–22].

In the present study, the extrinsic EAA agonist, aspartate, and antagonist, ketamine, showed different effects on hypoxic preconditioning. T_s in each hypoxic run and survival time in hypobaric chambers are both in the order of ASP < NS < KET. This result indicates that the activation of ionotropic NMDA receptors is harmful while the suppression of ionotropic NMDA receptors is beneficial to the formation of hypoxic preconditioning.

Ketamine, a PCP derivative, is an NMDA-noncompetitive antagonist and has been proved by extensive studies to be a neuroprotective substance [23–26]. Ketamine is able to combine with the PCP site in the NMDA receptor complex, to interfere with the combination of EAAs with NMDA receptors and to block the opening of the iron channel, thus alleviating the Ca^{2+} influx and neuronal damage induced.

In preconditioning, after the 4th hypoxic run, the whole brain and different brain regions of mice suffering from longer and severer hypoxia should exhibit increased EAA levels if no self- or other protective action is involved. However, in the present study, no increase in the concentrations of aspartate and glutamate was shown when the number of exposure runs was increased; on the contrary, the content of aspartate and glutamate in the whole brain, telencephalon and hippocampus was decreased, as well as that of glutamate in the cerebellum. Especially glutamate in the hippocampal region vulnerable to hypoxia decreased to normal levels. Besides, in other regions, the content remained at the same level as in hypoxic run 1 instead of increasing. This indicates that in preconditioning, degradation and/or inactivation of EAAs might be beneficial to the tolerance of mice to hypoxia, possibly as one of the self-protective mechanisms in preconditioning.

Acknowledgments

This project was supported by the National Natural Science Foundation of China (No. 3967027) and the Municipal Natural Science Foundation of Beijing (No. 7962009). This study was completed at the Department of Neurobiology of the Capital University of Medical Sciences. We highly appreciate the technical support given by Prof. Zhao-Hui Zeng of the Institute of Instrumental Analysis.

References

1 Graham SH, Shiraishi K, Panter SS, Simon RP, Faden AI: Changes in extracellular amino acid neurotransmitters produced by focal cerebral ischemia. Neurosci Lett 1990;110: 124–130.

2 Pellegrini-Giampietro DE, Cherici G, Alesiani M, Carlu V, Moroni F: Excitatory amino acid release from rat hippocampal slices as a consequence of free-radical formation. J Neurochem 1988;51:1960–1963.

3 Benveniste H, Horgensen MB, Sandberg M, Christensen T, Hagberg H, Diemer NH: Ischemic damage in hippocampal CA1 is dependent on glutamate release and intact innervation from CA3. J Cereb Blood Flow Metab 1989;9:629–639.

4 Mitan A, Kataoka K: Critical levels of glutamate extracellular glutamate-mediating gerbil hippocampal delayed neuronal death during hypothermia: Brain microdialysis study. Neuroscience 1991;42:661–670.

5 Korf J, Klein HC, Venema K, Postema F: Increases in striatal and hippocampal impedance and extracellular levels of amino acids by cardiac arrest in freely moving rats. J Neurochem 1988;50:1087–1096.

6 Rothman SM, Olney JW: Glutamate and the pathophysiology of hypoxic-ischemic brain damage. Ann Neurol 1986;19:105–111.

7 Choi DW, Rothman SM: The role of glutamate neurotoxicity in hypoxic-ischemic neuronal death. Annu Rev Neurosci 1991;13:172–182.

8 Lu GW, Ding DW, Shi MT: Acute adaptation of mice to hypoxic hypoxia. Biol Signals Recept 1999;8: 247–255.

9 Takagi K, Ginsberg MD, Globus MY, Dietrich WD, Martinez E, Kraydieh S, Busto R: Changes in amino acid neurotransmitters and cerebral blood flow in the ischemic penumbral region following middle cerebral artery occlusion in the rat: Correlation with histopathology. J Cereb Blood Flow Metab 1993;13: 575–585.

10 Watkins JC, Olverman HJ: Agonists and antagonists for excitatory amino acid receptors. Trends Neurosci 1987;10:265–272.

11 Soommer B, Seegurg PH: Glutamate receptor channels: Novel properties and new clones. Trends Pharmacol Sci 1992;13:291–296.

12 Choi DW, Kno NY, Peter S: Pharmacology of glutamate neurotoxicity in cortical cell culture: Attenuation by NMDA antagonist. J Neurosci 1988;8:185–186.

13 Raley-Susman KM, Lipton P: In vitro ischemia and protein synthesis in the rat hippocampal slice: The role of calcium and NMDA receptor activation. Brain Res 1990;525:27–38.
14 Choi DW: Excitotoxic cell death. J Neurobiol 1992;23:1261–1276.
15 Siesjo BK: Historical overview. Calcium, ischemia, and death of brain cells. Ann NY Acad Sci 1988;522: 638–661.
16 MacDermott AB, Mayer ML, Westbrook GL, Smith SJ, Barker JL: NMDA receptor activation increases cytoplasmic calcium concentration in cultured spinal cord neurones. Nature 1986;321:519–522.
17 Skadeozek F, Recasens M, Bockaert J: A new mechanism for glutamate receptor action, phosphoinositide hydrolysis. Trends Neurosci 1988; 11:545–549.
18 Hogg N, Darley-Usmar VM, Wilson MT, Moncada S: Production of hydroxyl radicals from the simultaneous generation of superoxide and nitric oxide. Biochem J 1992;281: 419–424.
19 Buisson A, Margaill I, Callebert J, Plotkine M, Boulu RG: Mechanisms involved in the neuroprotective activity of a nitric oxide synthase inhibitor during focal cerebral ischemia. J Neurochem 1993;61:690–696.
20 Moncada S, Higgs A: The *L*-argine-nitric oxide pathway. N Engl J Med 1993;329:2002–2012.
21 Kozniewska E, Roberts TP, Tsuura M, Mintorovitch J, Moseley ME, Kucharczyk J: NG-nitro-*L*-arginine delays the development of brain injury during focal ischemia in rats. Stroke 1995;26:282–288.
22 Stamler SS, Singel DJ, Loscalzo J: Biochemistry of nitric oxide and its redox-activated forms. Science 1989;258:1898–1902.
23 Marcoux FW, Goodrich JE, Dominick MA: Ketamine prevents ischemic neuronal injury. Brain Res 1988;452:329–335.
24 Church J, Zeman S, Lodge D: The neuroprotective function of ketamine and MK-801 after transient ischemic ischemia in rats. Anesthesiology 1988;69:702–709.
25 Rothman SM, Thurston JH, Hauhart RE, Clark GD, Solomon JS: Ketamine protects hippocampal neurons from anoxia in vitro. Neuroscience 1987;21:673–678.
26 Pohorecki R, Becker GL, Reilly PJ, Landers DF: Ischemic brain injury in vitro: Protective effects of NMDA receptor antagonists and calmidazolium. Brain Res 1990; 528:133–137.

Biological Signals and Receptors

Biol Signals Recept 1999;8:275–280

Received: October 15, 1998
Accepted: October 30, 1998

Changes of Adenosine and Its A_1 Receptor in Hypoxic Preconditioning

Wei-Li Zhang[a] Guo-Wei Lu[b]

[a]Beijing Neurosurgical Institute, and [b]Department of Neurobiology, Capital University of Medical Sciences, Beijing, China

Key Words
Hypoxia · Hypoxic preconditioning · Adenosine · Adenosine receptor

Abstract
Effects of hypoxic preconditioning on adenosine (ADO) and its A_1 receptor were studied in Kunming mice. The ADO content and its metabolites in the brain were measured by a specific enzymatic method; a radioligand binding method was used to study the ADO A_1 receptor. The ADO content of the hippocampus in group C (exposure to 4 runs of hypoxia) was markedly higher than that in group A (control, without exposure to hypoxia and B (exposure to 1 run of hypoxia), showing that the ADO content could be cumulatively increased in the hippocampus, which was more sensitive to ischemia and hypoxia, during acute and repeated exposure to hypoxia. A_1 receptor density in group C was significantly lower than in group A and no difference was seen between groups B and C; A_1 receptor affinity in the hippocampus, pons and medula oblongata in group C was significantly higher than in group A, implying that during hypoxic preconditioning there might be some mechanisms preventing A_1 receptor density from decreasing further and making A_1 receptor affinity increase in some brain regions. These results indicate that cumulatively increased ADO in the hippocampus via A_1 receptor may play a neuroprotective role in the CNS as an inhibitory neuromodulator and thus contribute to the formation and development of acute hypoxic adaptation or tolerance.

Introduction

Adenosine (ADO) is the metabolic product of ATP and may play many physiological roles in the CNS via its receptors. ADO is rec-

KARGER

Fax + 41 61 306 12 34
E-Mail karger@karger.ch
www.karger.com

1422–4933/99/0085–0275$17.50/0

Accessible online at:
http://BioMedNet.com/karger

Wei-Li Zhang
Beijing Neurosurgical Institute
Chong Wen District Tianton Xili No. 6
Beijing 100050 (China)

ognized as an inhibitory neuromodulator playing a neuroprotective role in the CNS [1]. A lot of work has been done on the relation between ADO and ischemia or hypoxia and some of it has touched the cellular and molecular level, but little is known about its role in hypoxic preconditioning [2]. The effects of ADO, N^6-cyclohexyladenosine (CHA), a selective ADO A_1 receptor agonist, and aminotheophylline (AMT), a receptor antagonist, were examined during acute and repeated exposure to hypoxia, and survival time of the animals in a hypobaric chamber (PO_2 = 2.7 kPa) was tested. The tolerance and survival time were significantly prolonged by CHA and shortened by AMT. These results indicate that activation of the ADO A_1 receptor can significantly augment the animal's tolerance to hypoxia whereas blockade of ADO receptors is not benificial to the development of hypoxia adaptation. In order to explore the mechanism underlying hypoxic tolerance, the contents of ADO and its metabolites and ADO A_1 receptor in the brains of mice during acute repeated exposure to hypoxia were measured in the present study.

Materials and Methods

Preparation of the Animal Model [3]

Adult Kunming mice of either sex weighing between 19 and 22 g were used in the present study. Experiments were conducted on groups A (control, without hypoxic exposure), B (exposure to 1 run of hypoxia) and C (exposure to 4 runs of hypoxia). Room temperature was at 18–22 °C. The mouse was weighed, and put into a sealed bottle with a volume of about 150 ml and full of fresh air. When gasping was noted, the mouse was immediately taken out and transferred into another identical bottle. This procedure was repeated 4 times. The animals in each group were decapitated following the last exposure. Their brains were rapidly removed, placed on an ice-cold glass plate, the hippocampus, mesencephalon, diencephalon, pons, cerebellum and medulla oblongata were removed and immediately frozen in liquid nitrogen.

Assay of ADO and Its Metabolites [4]

The brains were weighed, homogenized (6 ml 0.6 *M* $HClO_4$ was added to the whole brain, and 3 ml of 0.6 *M* $HClO_4$ to each region), and centrifuged at 2 °C, 24,000 *g* for 30 min. The supernatant was neutralized by 5 *M* K_2CO_3 to pH 7.4, and centrifuged at 2 °C, 24,000 *g* for 25 min. The supernatant thus obtained was suspended with ½ volume Tris-HCl buffer containing 3 *M* K_2HPO_4 and 3 *M* EDTA. Then ADO and its metabolites were measured with a UV-3000 spectrophotometer (Shimadzu, Japan). Xanthine oxidase (0.08 U), 5′-nucleoside phosphorylase (0.04 U) and ADO deaminase (0.08 U) (Boehringer Mannheim, Indianapolis, Ind., USA) were added to the above suspensions, and the absorption curves (ΔE_{292}) for hypoxanthine (HX), inosine INO and ADO contents obtained. The HX, INO and ADO contents (μM/mg tissue) were measured according to a standard curve.

Radioreceptor Assays [5]

Crude synaptic membrane fractions were prepared from different brain regions and suspended in 40 vol of 50 m*M* Tris-HCl buffer (pH 7.4), centrifuged at 50,000 *g* for 30 min. These washing procedures were repeated three times, and the final pellets were suspended in 8 vol of 0.32 *M* sucrose, frozen at −80 °C until use. All the above procedures were carried out at 4 °C. On the day of the experiment, frozen suspensions were thawed at room temperature and the thawed suspensions were washed three times with 40 vol of 50 m*M* Tris-HCl buffer (pH 7.4). The suspensions were then incubated with ADO deaminase (2 U/ml) in a rolling incubator at 37 °C for 45 min, and terminated by the addition of 15 ml of ice-cold buffer followed by centrifugation as mentioned above. The final pellets were resuspended to a final concentration of 1–2 mg/ml protein for the binding assays. Protein content was determined using the BCA protein assay reagents (Pierce Chemical Co., Rockford, Ill., USA) [6]. After pretreatment, 100 µl of the membrane suspensions (about 0.1–0.2 mg) were incubated at room temperature with 0–40 n*M* N^6-cyclohexyl ^3H adenosine (^3H-CHA, 34.4 Ci/m*M*, New England Nuclear, Boston, Mass., USA) for 60 min in 1 ml of 50 m*M* Tris-HCl buffer (pH 7.4). Incubation was terminated by the addition of 5 ml of ice-cold buffer at 2 °C and subsequent filtration through a Whatman GF/B glass fiber filter under a constant vacuum of 2.0 kPa. The filter was rinsed four times with 5 ml of ice-cold buffer at 2 °C within 10 s and radioactivity retained on the filter was measured with a liquid scintillation spectrometer (Beckman 5801, USA). Nonspecific binding was determined by unlabeled CHA (1 μM, Sigma, St. Louis, Mo., USA).

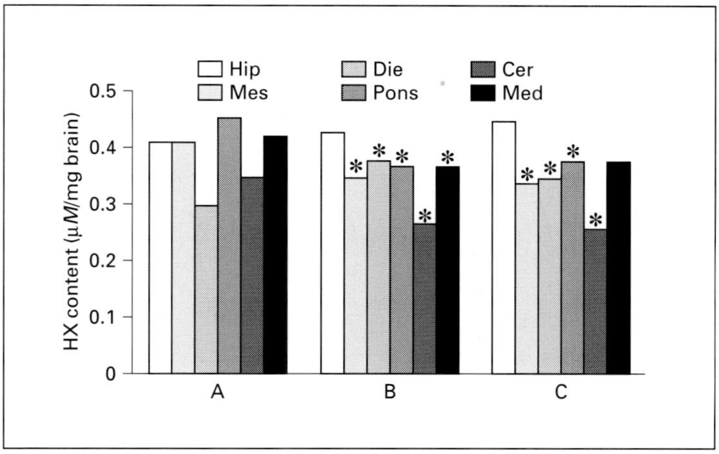

Fig. 1. Content of HX in different regions of mouse brain (mean ± SE). * $p < 0.05$ vs. group A. Hip = Hippocampus; Mes = mesencephalon; Die = diencephalon; Cer = cerebellum; Med = medulla oblongata.

Table 1. Contents of ADO and its metabolites in the mouse whole brain (μ*M*/mg brain, mean ± SE, n = 20)

Group	HX	INO	ADO
A	0.042 ± 0.003	0.024 ± 0.004	0.037 ± 0.004
B	0.068 ± 0.006*	0.063 ± 0.016*	0.056 ± 0.003**
C	0.074 ± 0.006**	0.071 ± 0.006*	0.122 ± 0.014**, °°

* $p < 0.05$, ** $p < 0.01$ vs. group A. °° $p < 0.01$ vs. group B.

Specific binding was calculated as the difference between total and nonspecific binding. The affinity constant K_d and total number of binding sites (B_{max}) values were determined using Scatchard analysis.

Statistical Analysis

Data were expressed as mean ± SE and tested for significant differences between various groups of animals by one-way analysis of variance (ANOVA) and Duncan's multiple-comparison test.

Results

Contents of ADO and Its Metabolites in Mouse Whole Brain

Contents of ADO, INO and HX significantly increased in groups B and C, and ADO content in group C was significantly higher than in group B (table 1).

Contents of ADO and Its Metabolites in Different Regions of Mouse Brain

Compared with the different brain regions in group A, except for the hippocampus in group B and the hippocampus, medula oblongata in group C, HX content in other brain regions was markedly changed (fig. 1). INO content of the hippocampus, diencephalon and medula oblongata in group B and INO content of the cerebellum and medulla oblongata in group C were markedly changed (fig. 2). ADO content of the hippocampus, mesencephalon, diencephalon in group B and, except for the cerebellum in group C, was significantly increased. ADO content of the hippocampus in group C was significantly higher than in group B (fig. 3).

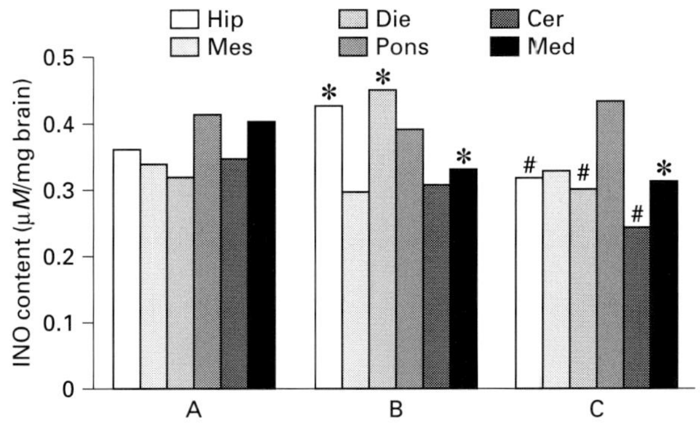

Fig. 2. Content of INO in different regions of mouse brain (mean ± SE). * $p < 0.05$ vs. group A. # $p < 0.05$ vs. group B. Abbreviations, as in figure 1.

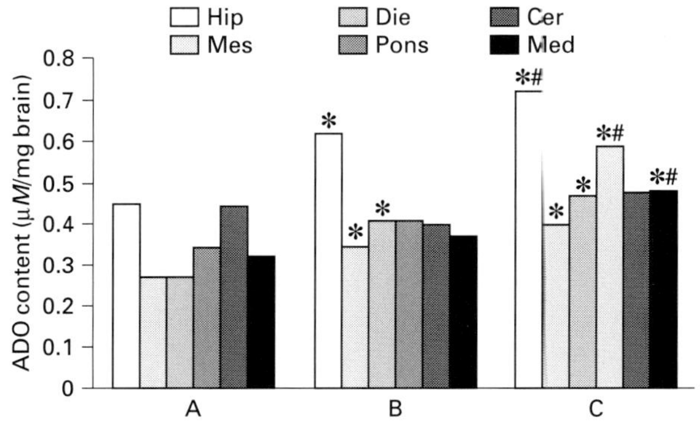

Fig. 3. Content of ADO in different regions of mouse brain (mean ± SE). * $p < 0.05$ vs. group A, # $p < 0.05$ vs. group B. Abbreviations, as in figure 1.

Table 2. Value of K_d and B_{max} of ADO A_1 receptor in different brain regions of groups A, B and C (mean ± SE, n = 10)

Region	K_d, n*M*			B_{max}, pmol/mg protein		
	A	B	C	A	B	C
Hip	7.07±0.02	7.05±0.03	6.05±0.07*	9.02±0.02	6.84±0.06*	6.93±0.04*
Mes	7.04±0.02	7.03±0.03	7.01±0.03	6.47±0.03	5.21±0.06*	5.24±0.07*
Die	7.04±0.03	7.04±0.02	7.00±0.03	6.59±0.04	5.16±0.05*	5.13±0.08*
Pons	7.04±0.02	6.87±0.10	5.81±0.06*	7.14±0.05	5.37±0.08*	5.40±0.10*
Cer	7.03±0.02	7.02±0.03	7.00±0.04	10.77±0.20	8.26±0.08*	8.21±0.07*
Med	6.98±0.08	7.01±0.04	5.77±0.08*	8.27±0.06	6.31±0.10*	6.31±0.07*

* $p < 0.05$ vs. group A. Hip = Hippocampus; Mes = mesencephalon; Die = diencephalon; Cer = cerebellum; Med = medulla oblongata.

Changes of A_1 Receptor in Different Regions of Mouse Brain

A_1 receptor density of group B and C was significantly lower than that of group A, whereas no difference was seen between groups B and C. A_1 receptor affinity in the hippocampus, pons and medulla oblongata in group C was markedly higher than in group A and no difference was seen between groups A and B (table 2).

Discussion

The present study showed that the contents of ADO, INO and HX in whole mouse brains of groups exposed to hypoxia were significantly higher than in a control group not exposed to hypoxia. The major source of ADO is ATP which is metabolized intracellularly to ADO, and excess ADO is then transported out of the cell. Some ADO is metabolized into INO and HX by ADO deaminase and nucleoside phosphorylase. Thus the contents of ADO, INO and HX were markedly increased. Through repetitive exposure to hypoxia, the tolerance time was significantly prolonged [3], and the ADO level in the brain was markedly higher than in the group exposed to hypoxia for 1 run, while the levels of HX and INO did not differ between two hypoxia groups. These results indicate that some mechanism might inhibit ADO degradation under circumstances of acute and repeated exposure to hypoxia and ADO might thus accumulate. ADO exerts a number of actions that may reduce the extent of cell death. ADO could inhibit neuronal Ca^{2+} uptake and excitatory amino acid (glutamate and aspartate) release via A_1 receptors situated on the presynaptic membrane, inhibit adenylcyclase activity and cAMP release via A_1 animals situated on the postsynaptic membrane, and induce neuron membrane hyperpolarization which would decrease neuronal activities [7]. Xie et al. [8] have reported increased in excitatory amino acids in hypoxic preconditioned mice. It has also been reported that ATP can be formed from endogenous adenosine and that this metabolic regeneration leads to neuroprotection [9]. Recently, Ramkumar et al. [10] showed that ADO may enhance the activity of antioxidant enzymes, such as superoxide dismutase, via A_3 receptors and play a cytoprotective role during ischemia. Therefore, ADO accumulated in the brain through repetitive exposure to hypoxia facilitates adaptation to hypoxia.

In the present study, the contents of HX, INO and ADO of the group exposed to hypoxia were not found to be increased in all brain regions. Compared with the group exposed to hypoxia for 1 run, INO and HX contents in different regions were not increased cumulatively during acute hypoxia for 4 runs, while the ADO content in the hippocampus markedly increased. Certain regions of the brain (i.e., hippocampus) are particularly vulnerable to hypoxia or ischemia [11]. Via its A_1 receptor, accumulated adenosine is believed to inhibit the excess release of excitatory neurotransmitters, most likely glutamate and aspartate, and decrease their excitotoxicity, and thus attenuate the ischemia-induced neuronal damage.

The neuroprospective role of ADO during hypoxia is related to extracellular ADO metabolism, ADO receptor affinity and density. In particular, A_1 receptor density has an important effect on controlling the strength of ADO modulation in the brain [12]. The present study showed that A_1 receptor density in the group exposed to hypoxia was significantly lower than that in the nonexposed control group. This indicates that the number of A_1 receptors would markedly decrease and be downregulated following hypoxia, which is in agreement with the results described by Lee et al. [13]. However, A_1 receptor density was not decreased any further with the repetition and prolongation of exposure to hypoxia. This indicates that the increase in endogenous ADO may limit the activity-evoked membrane depolarization and help maintain membrane stability, which protects A_1 receptors against further damage. Some changes may occur in the conformation of ADO A_1 receptors in the hippocampus, pons and medulla oblongata, and its affinity for its agonist CHA may thus be markedly increased during acute and repeated hypoxia. Through acute repeated hypoxia, animals develop acute adaptation to hypoxia and there may be some mechanisms to prevent a further decrease in the number of A_1 receptors and increase the affinity for A_1 receptors. All these changes may contribute to the neuroprotective role of ADO as a CNS neuromodulator via its receptors.

Acknowledgment

This work was supported by the National Natural Science Foundation of China (No. 39670271) and Beijing Natural Science Foundation (No. 7962009).

References

1 Rudolphi KA, Schubert P, Parkinson FE, Fredholm BB: Neuroprotective role of adenosine in cerebral ischemia. Trends Pharmacol Sci 1992;13:439–445.
2 Zhang WL, Lu GW: Effects of adenosine in hypoxia tolerance in mice repeatedly exposed to acute hypoxia. Basic Med Sci Clin 1996;16:69–71.
3 Lu GW, Ding DW, Shi MT: Acute adaptation of mice to hypoxic hypoxia. Biol Signals Recept 1999;8:247–255.
4 Sun JW, Wang SY, Lu LQ, Meng FY, Ding ZY: Changes of purine nucleoside contents in rabbit brain and cerebrospinal fluid during acute cerebral hypoxia. Chin J Pathophysiol 1993;9:613–615.
5 Bruns RF, Daly JW, Snyder SH: Adenosine receptors in brain membranes: Binding of N^6-cyclohexyl [^{3}H] adenosine and 1,3-diethyl-8-[^{3}H] phenylxanthine. Proc Natl Acad Sci USA 1980;77:5547–5551.
6 Smith PK, Krohn RI, Hermonson GT: Measurement of protein using bicinchoninic acid. Anal Biochem 1985;150:76–85.
7 Corradetti R, Conto GL, Moroni F, Passani MB, Pepeu G: Adenosine dereases aspartate and glutamate release from rat hippocampal slices. Eur J Pharmacol 1984;104:19–21.
8 Xie JH, Lu GW, Hou YZ: Role of excitatory amino acids in hypoxic preconditioning. Biol Signals Recept 1999;8:267–274.
9 Deckert J, Gleiter CH: Adenosine – an endogenous neuroprotective metabolite and neuromodulator. J Neural Transm 1994;43(suppl):23–31.
10 Ramkumar V, Nie ZZ, Rybak LP, Maggirwar SB: Adenosine, antioxidant enzymes and cytoprotection. Trends Pharmacol Sci 1995;16:283–285.
11 Rothman SM, Olney JW: Excitotoxity and the NMDA receptor. Trends Neurosci 1987;10:299–302.
12 Lee KS, Redding M, Schubert P: Regulation of the strength of adenosine modulation in the hippocampus by a differential distribution of the density of A_1 receptors. Brain Res 1983;260:156–159.
13 Lee KS, Tetzlaff W, Kreatzberg GW: Rapid downregulation of hippocampal adenosine receptors following brief anoxia. Brain Res 1986;380:155–158.

Biological Signals and Receptors

Biol Signals Recept 1999;8:281–293

Received: November 3, 1998
Accepted: November 17, 1998

Hypoxia-Ischemia-Induced Apoptotic Cell Death Correlates with IGF-I mRNA Decrease in Neonatal Rat Brain

Teresa F. Clawson[a] Susan J. Vannucci[b] Guo-Ming Wang[a]
Lisa B. Seaman[b] Xian-Lin Yang[a] Wei-Hua Lee[a]

[a]Department of Pediatrics, Indiana University School of Medicine, Indianapolis, Ind., and
[b]Department of Pediatrics, College of Medicine, The Milton S. Hershey Medical Center, Pennsylvania State University, Hershey, Pa., USA

Key Words
Hypoxia-ischemia · Brain · Apoptosis · IGF-I

Abstract
Hypoxia-ischemia induces apoptotic and necrotic cell death, which results partially from persistent alterations in cellular energy homeostasis. Insulin-like growth factor I (IGF-I) is an anabolic pleiotrophic factor required by developing neurons for their optimal proliferation, differentiation, and survival. To determine how cell death and changes in IGF-I gene expression relate to the extent of hypoxia-ischemia, we evaluated the time course of apoptosis in a neonatal hypoxia-ischemia model in relation to the cellular distribution of IGF-I and IGFBP5 mRNA. Severe hypoxia-ischemia results in an immediate decrease in neuronal IGF-I and IGFBP5 mRNA. The decrease in neuronal IGF-I mRNA was concurrent with an increase in the number of apoptotic cells. It is conceivable that the immediate decrease in IGF-I gene expression may contribute to the impending neuronal death and selective vulnerability of myelinogenesis during the perinatal period.

Introduction

Perinatal hypoxia-ischemia severe enough to produce permanent brain damage is associated with both widespread and selective neuronal necrosis. Recent evidence shows that hypoxia-ischemia also induces apoptotic cell death [1–3], as evidenced by morphological changes, internucleosomal DNA cleavage and DNA fragmentation [4]. Apoptosis is an active selective process that eliminates extraneous or dangerous cells [5]. After a hypoxic-ischemic insult, an increased number of neurons undergo apoptosis or necrosis [6, 7], with variations of each according to cell type, state of differentiation and regional distribution

KARGER
Fax + 41 61 306 12 34
E-Mail karger@karger.ch
www.karger.com

Accessible online at:
http://BioMedNet.com/karger

Wei-Hua Lee, PhD, MD
Section of Neonatal-Perinatal Medicine, Department of Pediatrics
Indiana University School of Medicine, 699 West Drive, RR 208
Indianapolis, IN 46202-5119 (USA)
Tel. +1 (317) 274 4715, Fax +1 (317) 274 2065, E-Mail wlee@iupui.edu

[8]. The extent of apoptosis is proportional to the duration of the hypoxic-ischemic episode and the degree of high-energy phosphate depletion [6–8]. To date, the factors that initiate apoptosis following hypoxia-ischemia and the relationship between the duration of hypoxia-ischemia and the onset of apoptosis have not been defined.

Apoptosis may be initiated when an essential trophic factor declines below a threshold level [9, 10]. Insulin-like growth factor-I (IGF-I) is an anabolic neurotrophic factor and plays a regulatory role in cellular energy metabolism that is of key importance during hypoxic-ischemic insult [11]. Perinatal hypoxic-ischemic injury results in an immediate decrease in the expression of neuronal IGF-I and IGFBP5 in rat brains [11–14]. Interestingly, intraventricular infusion of IGF-I two hours post-ischemia ameliorates neuronal damage in rat and [14–17] sheep [18]. These observations suggest that a decrease in neuronal IGF-I is involved in the injury to the developing neurons [1, 12–14, 19, 20] and that providing IGF-I may prevent neuronal loss.

We hypothesize that the decrease in neuronal IGF-I after a hypoxic-ischemic insult contributes to the increase in apoptosis. To test this hypothesis, we induced cerebral hypoxia-ischemia in postnatal day 7 rats using a well-established, reproducible rat model for perinatal asphyxial encephalopathy [21]. In this model, DNA fragmentation has been used as an indicator of apoptotic cell death, based on the correlation between in situ labeling of 3′-OH ends of DNA and internucleosomal DNA cleavage [4]. Following increasing lengths of hypoxia-ischemia, we used adjacent sections to study IGF-I and IGFBP5 gene expression by in situ hybridization and apoptosis by in situ DNA fragmentation analysis. In addition, we compared the relationship between the duration of hypoxic-ischemic insult, changes in IGF-I and IGFBP5, and neuronal demise.

Methods

Hypoxia-Ischemia Model

Pregnant Wistar rats (Charles River) were housed in individual cages and fed standard laboratory chow ad libitum. Offspring were delivered vaginally, and litter size was adjusted to 10 pups/litter on the day of delivery and remained with the dam until the day of experimentation. Hypoxia-ischemia was induced in 7-day-old rat pups as previously described [21], with minor modifications. Day 7 rats were used, since the maturity of their brains is roughly comparable to that of a 32- to 34-week gestation human fetus or newborn infant [21]. Their cerebral cortical layering is completed, the germinal matrix is involuting and white matter is beginning to myelinate [22]. Before exposure to hypoxia (8% O_2/92% N_2), pups were placed in a container immersed in a 37 °C water bath for 20 min followed by 60, 90, 120 or 150 min of exposure to hypoxia. Preliminary studies demonstrated that this period of prewarming produced a more uniform degree of damage in littermates, but required a reduction in the hypoxic exposure to ensure survival. Unilateral common carotid artery ligation combined with 8% oxygen produces brain damage predominantly in the territory of the middle cerebral artery of the cerebral hemisphere ipsilateral to the carotid artery occlusion [21]. Hypoxia-only animals were exposed to 8% oxygen for 150 min without any operative procedures. Damage does not usually occur in the hemisphere if only exposed to ischemia or hypoxia. Control animals were placed in the 37 °C water bath for 150 min and were not rendered hypoxic or ischemic. All rat pups were then returned to their dams for 1, 24, or 72 h, at which times they were killed by decapitation, and the brains were removed and frozen in isopentane at –55 °C, and stored at –70 °C until sectioned at 16 µm thickness for in situ hybridization and immunocytochemical analysis. For each animal, at least 4 sections were analyzed for each experiment.

In situ Hybridization

Rat IGF-I and IGFBP5 subclones were used for the synthesis of cRNA probes as described previously [23]. Briefly, ^{35}S-labeled antisense riboprobes were synthesized in 10 µl of reaction mixture containing 100 µCi each of ^{35}S-CTP and ^{35}S-UTP (New England Nuclear), 10 m*M* NaCl, 6 m*M* $MgCl_2$, 40 m*M* Tris (pH 7.5), 2 m*M* spermidine, 10 m*M* dithiothreitol (DTT), 500 µ*M* each unlabeled ATP and GTP, 25 µ*M* each unlabeled UTP and CTP, 1 µg of linearized template, 15 U of the appropriate polymerase (BRL) and 15 U of RNasin (Promega). The reaction was incubated at

42 °C for 60 min, after which the DNA template was removed by digestion with DNase I. Prior to hybridization, tissue sections were warmed to 25 °C, fixed in 4% formaldehyde, and acetylated in 0.25% acetic anhydride, 0.1 *M* triethanolamine hydrochloride, 0.9% NaCl. Tissue was dehydrated through an ethanol gradient, delipidated in chloroform, rehydrated, and air-dried. ^{35}S-labeled cRNA probes were added to fresh hybridization buffer (10^7 cpm/ml) composed of 50% formamide, 0.3 *M* NaCl, 20 m*M* Tris-HCl (pH 8), 5 m*M* EDTA, 500 μg of tRNA/ml, 10% dextran sulfate, 10 m*M* DTT, and 0.02% each of BSA, Ficoll, and polyvinylpyrolidone. Hybridization buffer was added to sections, which were then covered with glass coverslips and placed in humidified chambers overnight (14 h) at 55 °C. Afterwards, slides were washed several times in 4 × saline-sodium citrate (SSC) to remove coverslips and hybridization buffer, dehydrated, and immersed in 0.3 *M* NaCl, 50% formamide, 20 m*M* Tris-HCl, 1 m*M* EDTA at 60 °C for 15 min. Sections were then treated with RNase A (20 μg/ml; Boehringer Mannheim, Indianapolis, Ind., USA) for 30 min at 37 °C and passed through graded salt solutions, followed by a 15-min wash in 0.1 × SSC at 50 °C. Slides were dehydrated, air-dried, and apposed to Hyperfilm-beta Max (Amersham) for 1–5 days, and then dipped in Kodak NTB3 nuclear emulsion, stored with desiccant at 4 °C for 3–15 days, developed, and stained with hematoxylin and eosin for microscopic evaluation. The level of nonspecific signal was determined by hybridization of parallel tissue sections with a sense probe synthesized from the IGFR-I clone since IGFR-I has the most ubiquitous presence of all IGF system genes. Scoring of changes in IGF-I mRNA expression were performed by an individual blinded to the results of apoptosis labeling.

Apoptosis Labeling

Analysis of DNA fragmentation in tissue sections was carried out using a nonradioactive approach, as described previously [24] with the following modifications. Fresh frozen sections were hydrated and treated with proteinase K (1 μg/ml in 20 m*M* Tris and 2 m*M* $CaCl_2$, pH 7.4) for 30 min at 37 °C in a humidified chamber, followed by three washes in Tris buffer (100 m*M* Tris and 150 m*M* NaCl, pH 7.5). Tissue sections were first incubated in terminal transferase buffer (200 m*M* potassium cacodylate, 25 m*M* Tris, 0.25 mg/ml BSA, and 5 m*M* $CoCl_2$, pH 6.6) for 10 min at room temperature. Afterwards, terminal transferase (0.3 U/μl; Boehringer Mannheim), digoxigenin-ddUTP (dig-ddUTP, 5 μ*M*; Boehringer Mannheim), and ddATP (45 μ*M*; Pharmacia, Uppsala, Sweden) were added in fresh buffer and incubated with tissue sections at 37 °C in a humidified chamber for 1 h. After one wash in Tris buffer and two washes in PBS, the sections were incubated with blocking buffer (5% normal rabbit serum in PBS, and 0.5% (w/v) blocking reagent; Boehringer Mannheim) for 30 min at room temperature before the addition of antidigoxigenin antibody (Boehringer Mannheim, 1:1,000 in 0.5% (w/v) blocking reagent, 5% normal rabbit serum, 1% BSA and 0.5% Triton X-100 in PBS). The sections were incubated at room temperature overnight in a humidified chamber, then washed three times in 0.1 *M* PBS containing 3% normal rabbit serum and 0.5% Triton X-100, and were incubated with rabbit antisheep biotinylated IgG (1:100 in PBS, 0.5% Triton) at room temperature for 1 h. The slides were again washed three times in 0.1 *M* PBS with 3% normal rabbit serum and 0.5% Triton X-100 preceding and following treatment with 0.5% H_2O_2 in absolute methanol for 10 min. Sections were incubated with avidin-biotin complex (1:50) in PBS containing 0.5% Triton X-100 for 1 h and washed twice in PBS. 3,3′-Diaminobenzidin (DAB) was added to develop color reaction for 2–10 min followed by PBS washes. Counterstaining was performed with 0.5% cresyl violet. Tissue sections were then dehydrated in graded alcohol and coverslipped.

Immunocytochemistry

Immunocytochemistry was performed on tissue sections adjacent to those used for in situ hybridization studies, to identify reactive astrocytes. A biotin-avidin-horseradish peroxidase method was used, employing a monoclonal antibody against glial fibrillary acidic protein (GFAP). After fixation in 4% formaldehyde fixative and blocking in 10% normal goat serum, tissue sections were incubated with a monoclonal antibody against GFAP (1:5, Boehringer Mannheim). Then, tissue sections were treated with biotinylated horse anti-mouse serum (1:200) for 2 h followed by a 45-min incubation with streptavidin-peroxidase conjugate. The antigen-antibody complex was visualized by incubation with DAB.

Quantification and Statistics

Cells stained positive for DNA cleavage were counted using photographs taken with a 40 × objective. Areas of analysis were selected from regions that demonstrated the most injury, such as cerebral cortex and thalamus that receive middle cerebral artery supply, as well as, the CA1 and CA2 regions of the hippocampus. Since there were multiple tissue sections on each slide, three areas each of cortex, hippocampus, and thalamus were photographed and counted on the first three tissue sections per slide, resulting in nine

Table 1. Apoptosis, IGF-I and IGFBP5 mRNA in hypoxic-ischemic injury

Duration of hypoxia-ischemia intervals	Following hypoxic-ischemic injury			Duration of hypoxia-ischemia intervals	Following hypoxic-ischemic injury		
	1 h	24 h	72 h		1 h	24 h	72 h
60 min				*150 min**			
Apoptotic cells	0	31 ± 4	42 ± 3	Apoptotic cells	110 ± 7	85 ± 5	97 ± 4
IGF-I	0	0	+++	IGF-I	–	–––	++++
IGFBP5	0	0	+++	IGFBP5	––	–––	+++
90 min				*150 min of hypoxia-only*			
Apoptotic cells	0	37 ± 7	47 ± 6	Apoptotic cells	0	0	0
IGF-I	0	0	+++	IGF-I	0	0	0
IGFBP5	0	0	+	IGFBP5	0	0	0
*120 min**				*Control*			
Apoptotic cells	0	73 ± 8	104 ± 7	Apoptotic cells	0	0	0
IGF-I	0	–,––	++++	IGF-I	0	0	0
IGFBP5	0	–––	++	IGFBP5	0	0	0

* $p < 0.05$ compared to shorter hypoxic-ischemic intervals.

The number of apoptotic cells represents the mean number of apoptotic cells counted in nine 40 × objective fields, three each from cortex, thalamus and hippocampus (see details in Methods section). In the same areas, IGF-I mRNA was scored compared to the contralateral side (approximate number of silver grains/cell: ––– = 5–20; –– = 15–30; – = 20–40; 0 = 40–60; + = 60–100; ++ = 90–170; +++ = 150–200; ++++ = 200–250). With increasing duration of hypoxic-ischemic exposure, apoptotic cell numbers increased, and peaked earlier in the recovery phase. Within 24 h following 120 min, and within 1 h following 150 min of hypoxia-ischemia, a decrease in IGF-I mRNA was seen in neurons. By 72 h of recovery, the cellular levels of IGF-I mRNA increased in astrocytes following all intervals of hypoxia-ischemia. IGFBP5 mRNA paralleled the changes in IGF-I mRNA. Neither apoptosis nor the pattern of IGF-I mRNA changed in animals exposed to 150 min of hypoxia-only in control animals, or on the contralateral side of injury.

areas of cortex, hippocampus, and thalamus, respectively. The extent of apoptosis in the hemisphere ipsilateral to the ligation was compared with the contralateral hemisphere. An individual blinded to the results of the IGF-I mRNA data performed the counts. Groups were compared by the Mann-Whitney test with a 2-tailed p value, comparing the median numbers of apoptotic cells for different times of ischemia.

Results

Apoptosis

The onset of apoptosis, as demonstrated by DNA cleavage, was noted within 1 h of recovery following 150 min of hypoxia-ischemia, and within 24 h following all intervals of hypoxia-ischemia less than 150 min (fig. 1). In general, the longer the hypoxic-ischemic interval, the earlier the peak number of apoptot-

Fig. 1. DNA cleavage following increasing hypoxia. Following left carotid artery ligation, D7 rats were exposed to 8% oxygen for 60 (**B**), 120 (**C**) and 150 (**D**) minutes and allowed to recover for 24 h. DNA cleavage was detected with DNA 3′-end labeling (brown staining) and sections were then counterstained with cresyl violet. **A** Normal morphology of parietal cortex where no cells stained positive for DNA cleavage. With increasing duration of hypoxic-ischemic exposure, the number of cells stained positive for DNA cleavage increased. Scale bar = 12.5 μM.

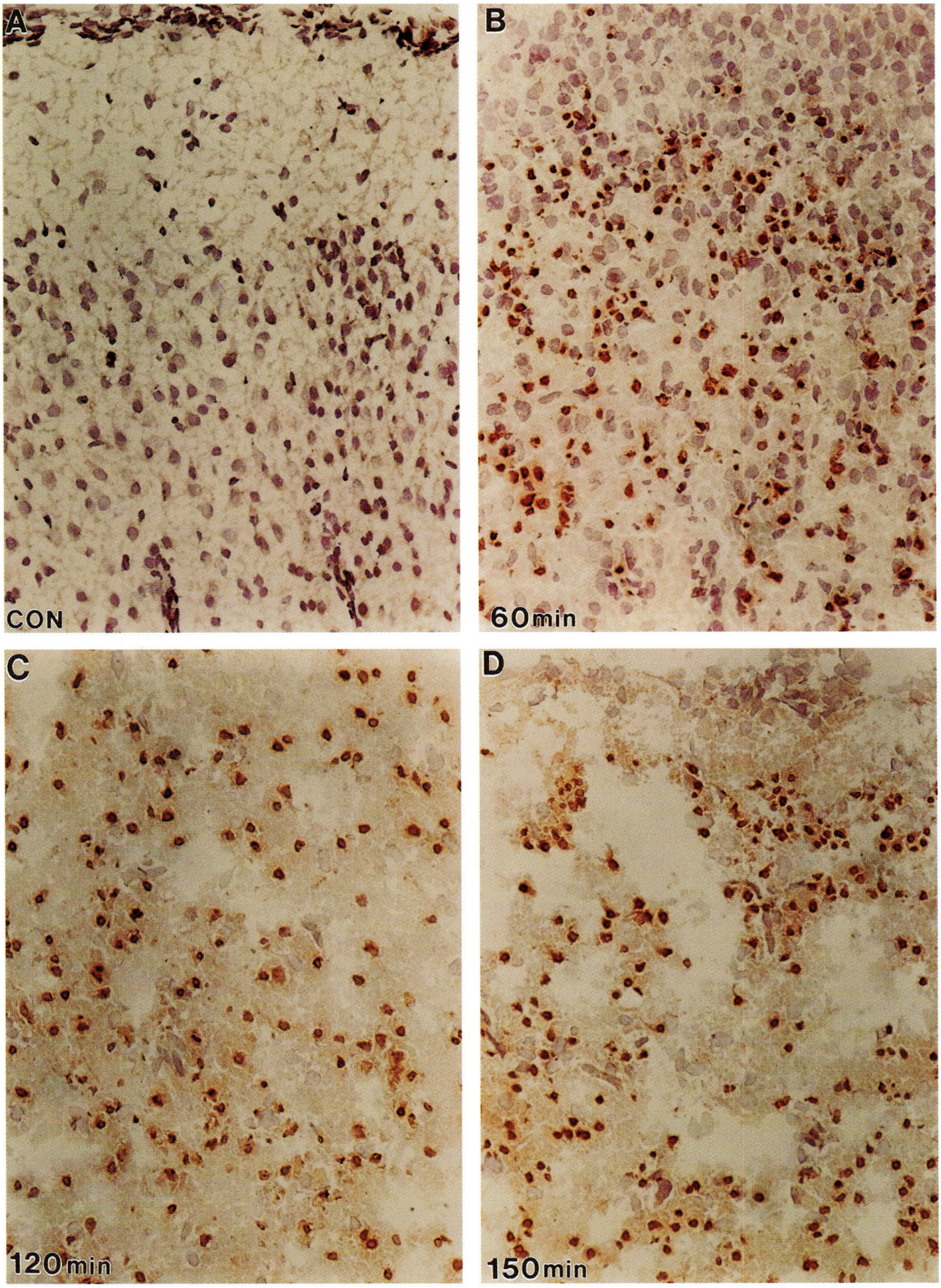
A
CON
B
60min
C
120min
D
150min

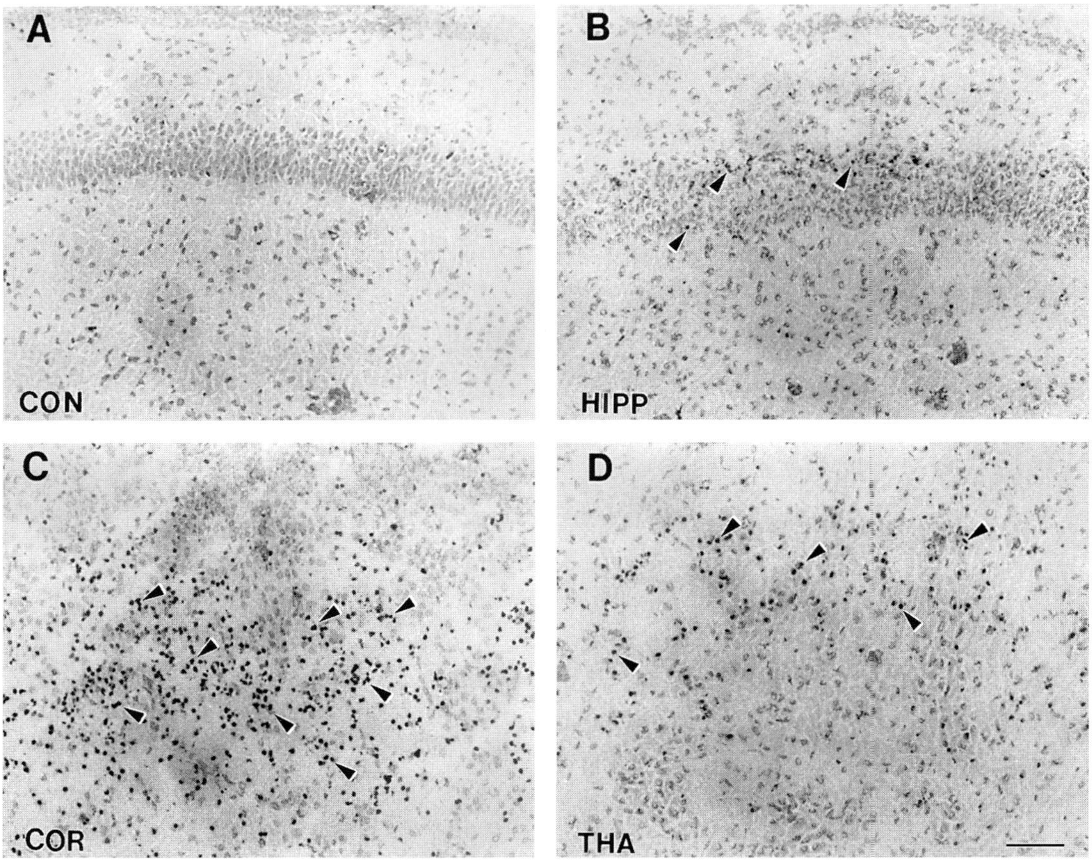

Fig. 2. Distribution of apoptotic cells in P7 rat brain. At 24 h following 60 min of hypoxia-ischemia, the greatest number of apoptotic cells was found in the cortex (**C**) as compared to the hippocampus (**B**) and the thalamus (**D**). While no apoptotic cells were found in the contralateral hippocampus (**A**), all apoptotic cells in the hippocampus were detected in the pyramidal cell layer (**B**). Scale bar = 12.5 μ*M*.

ic cells in the recovery phase: 1 h after 150 min of hypoxia-ischemia compared to 72 h after shorter hypoxic-ischemic intervals (table 1).

The extent of apoptosis was proportional to the duration of the hypoxic-ischemic episode. Following 60–90 min of hypoxia-ischemia, a significant number of cells showed DNA cleavage by 24 h of recovery (table 1). As the hypoxia time increased to 120 min, there was another significant increase in the number of apoptotic cells, which was further increased after 150 min of hypoxia-ischemia (table 1). Regional differences in response to hypoxia-ischemia existed, with the cortex most sensitive to the length of hypoxia-ischemia and the thalamus least sensitive (fig. 2). For example, an increase in apoptosis occurred with each 30-min increment in the cortex up to 120 min, whereas it was not until

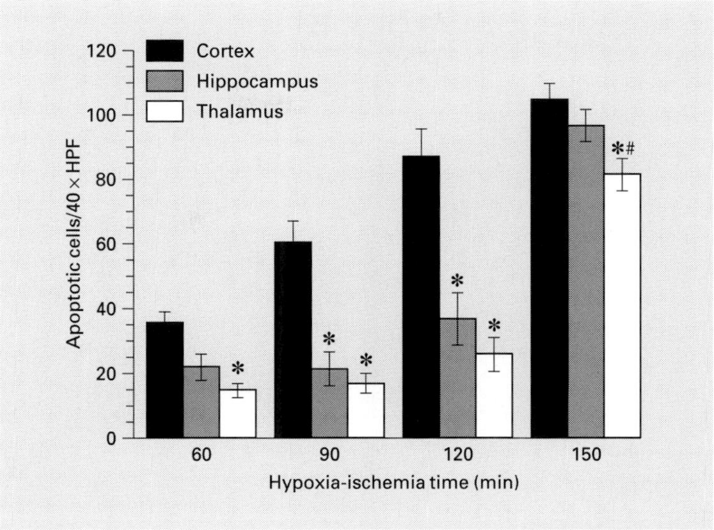

Fig. 3. Regional differences in apoptosis. Following hypoxic-ischemic injury, the number of apoptotic cells increased over hypoxia time, with greater increases found in the cortex. The increase in the apoptotic cells in the hippocampus and thalamus was comparable to that in the cortex only after 150 min of hypoxia-ischemia. * $p < 0.05$ compared to cortex, # $p < 0.05$ compared to hippocampus. Three animals were used for each time point and the number of apoptotic cells were counted in nine areas selected from each brain region.

150 min of hypoxia-ischemia that a significant increase occurred in the hippocampus or thalamus (fig. 3). Even after 150 min of hypoxia-ischemia, the number of apoptotic cells in the thalamus was less than the number in the cortex or hippocampus (fig. 3). Within the cerebral cortex, apoptotic cells distributed predominately in regions supplied by the middle cerebral artery.

No changes in apoptosis were noted in animals exposed to 150 min of hypoxia only, or in control animals (table 1).

IGF-I mRNA

A decrease in IGF-I mRNA in these neurons occurred with severe hypoxic-ischemic injury: within 24 h following 120 min of hypoxia-ischemia, and within 1 h following 150 min of hypoxia-ischemia (table 1). This hypoxia-ischemia-induced decrease in IGF-I mRNA occurred within large neurons, which normally express IGF-I mRNA (fig. 4A, D, 5A). By 72 h of recovery, IGF-I mRNA levels increased markedly in the thalamus, hippocampus, and cortical regions following all intervals of hypoxia-ischemia (table 1, fig. 3, 4). This increase of IGF-I mRNA expression occurred in reactive astrocytes as shown by their distribution similar to that of GFAP-positive astrocytes on adjacent sections (fig. 5). This astrocytic expression of IGF-I in the late recovery phase of hypoxic injury is consistent with previous studies [11].

The cellular distribution of IGF-I mRNA in large neurons of the contralateral hemisphere did not change over 72 h with hypoxia-ischemia at any length, nor was there a change in the IGF-I mRNA in control animals or in animals subjected to hypoxia only (table 1).

IGFBP5 mRNA

Changes in IGFBP5 mRNA paralleled the changes in IGF-I mRNA as previously described [16]. Similar to IGF-I, a decrease in neuronal expression of IGFBP5 mRNA was noted by 24 h following 120 min and by 1 h following 150 min of hypoxia-ischemia (table 1). An increase in the expression of IGFBP5 mRNA following all hypoxic-ischemic intervals was seen by 72 h (table 1). Like

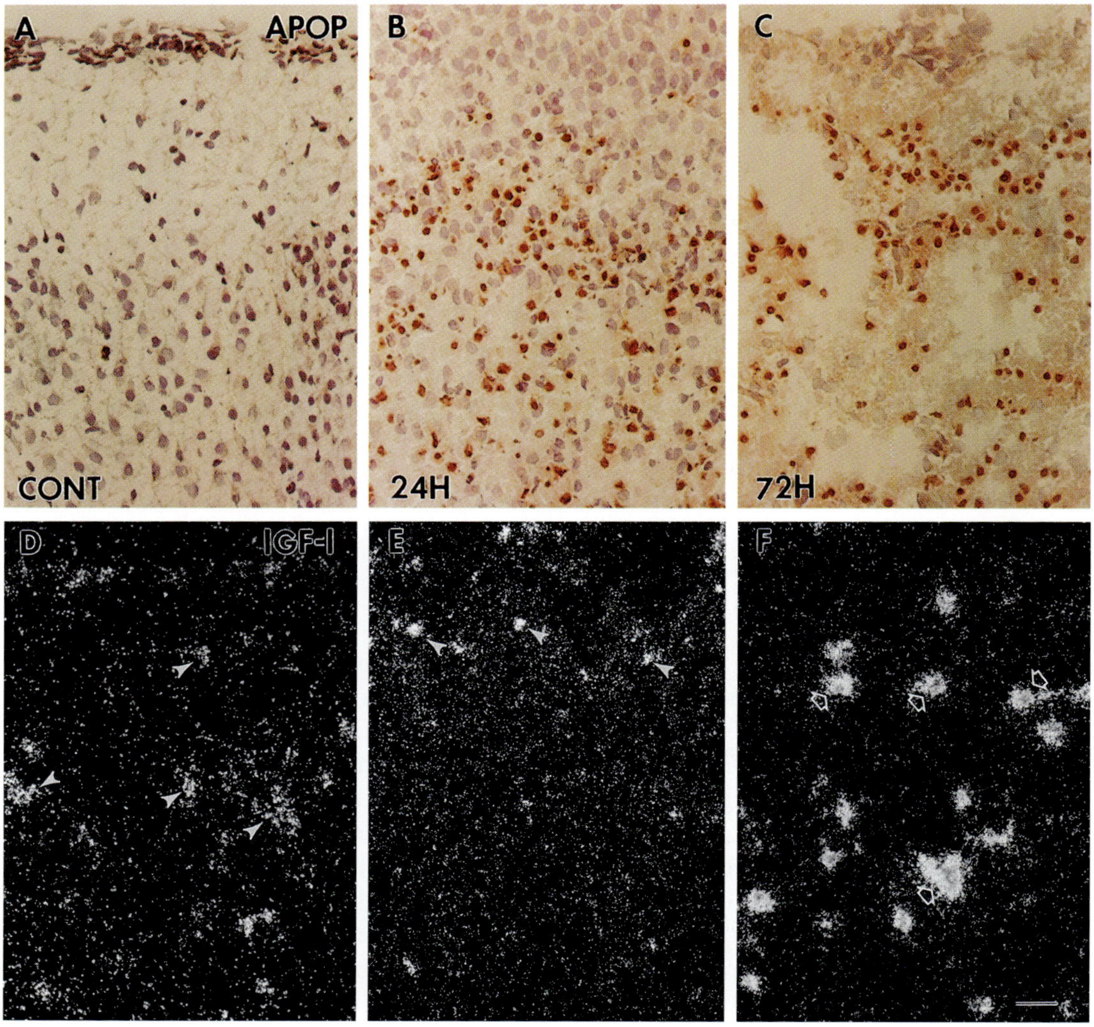

Fig. 4. Comparison of IGF-I mRNA level and number of apoptotic cells. At the first 24 h following hypoxia (120 min)-ischemia, the decreases in IGF-I mRNA levels (**E**) correlated with increases in the number of apoptotic cells (**B**, brown staining) on adjacent tissue sections. By 72 h of recovery, there was a columnar pattern seen in the ischemic cortex (**C**) and an increase in IGF-I mRNA in reactive astrocytes (**F**, see Results). The contralateral side to ligation is shown in **A** and **D**. Scale bar = 24 μm.

IGF-I, the cellular distribution IGFBP5 mRNA at 72 h of recovery resembles that of the distribution of GFAP-positive cells (fig. 5), and likely represents astrocytic expression.

Comparison of IGF-I and IGFBP5 mRNA and Apoptosis

During the first 24 h of recovery, the decrease in neuronal IGF-I and IGFBP5 mRNA following a severe hypoxic-ischemic insult of

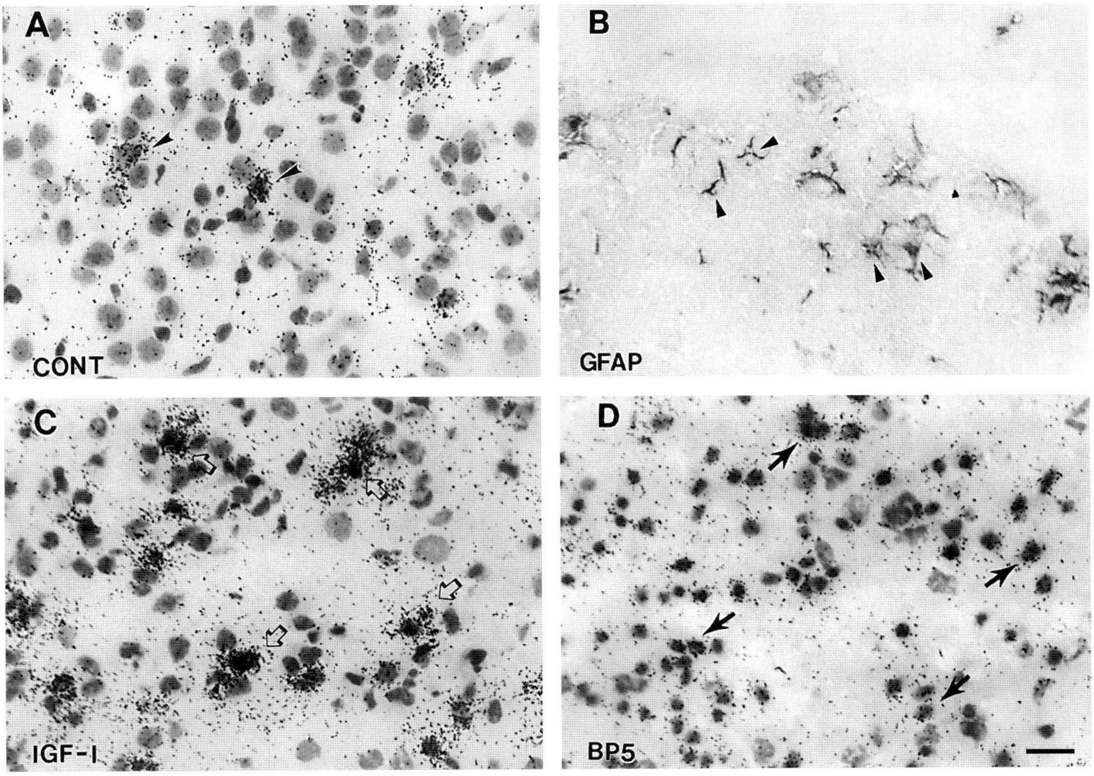

Fig. 5. Distribution of apoptotic cells, IGF-I mRNA, IGFBP5 mRNA, and GFAP positive cells on adjacent sections. At 72 h of recovery from hypoxia (120 min)-ischemia, there was an increased number of cells expressing IGF-I mRNA in the thalamus (**C**) compared to control (**A**). There was also an increase in the number of cells expressing IGFBP5 mRNA (**D**, control was not shown). On adjacent tissue sections, the distribution of IGF-I-expressing cells (**C**) was similar to that showing positive staining for GFAP (**B**, upper right). Scale bar = 12.5 μm.

120–150 min correlates with an increase in the number of apoptotic cells (table 1). At shorter hypoxic-ischemic intervals (60 or 90 min), no decreases in IGF-I or IGFBP5 mRNA were noted in neurons and there were relatively less apoptotic cells found (table 1). After a hypoxic-ischemic interval of 120 min, decreases in neuronal IGF-I and IGFBP5 mRNA occurred at 24 h of recovery concomitant with another significant increase in the number of apoptotic cells compared to earlier times (table 1). After 150 min of hypoxia-ischemia, decreases in IGF-I and IGFBP5 mRNA occurred within 1 h of recovery and persisted at 24 h of recovery. Also, apoptotic cells reached peak numbers within 1 h of recovery from 150 min of hypoxia-ischemia. Thus, the decreases in IGF-I and IGFBP5 mRNA following 150 min of hypoxia-ischemia also correlated with the increases in apoptosis.

Discussion

Perinatal hypoxia-ischemia induces necrosis as well as apoptosis in the brain [7, 8]. Apoptotic cells can be identified by the morphological changes such as cell shrinkage, condensation of chromatin and formation of apoptotic bodies as well as by DNA internucleosomal cleavage. In immature rodent brains, hypoxia-ischemia activates the apoptosis program within postischemic tissue [2, 6, 16, 22, 25–28]. This hypoxia-ischemia induced apoptosis may exacerbate the ongoing developmental cell death since the immature cells have high metabolic demand for growth and are therefore vulnerable to the ischemic insult [8]. This study intends to address the potential relationship between the extent of apoptotic cell death, demonstrated by DNA fragmentation in situ, and the level of neuronal IGF-I mRNA, shown by in situ hybridization.

The duration of the hypoxic-ischemic insult affected both the degree of apoptosis and the rapidity of its onset during the recovery period. Cells stained positive for apoptosis can be seen after 60 min of hypoxia-ischemia. As the hypoxia-ischemia prolonged to 120 min there was a dramatic increase in the number of apoptotic cells, which was further increased after 150 min of hypoxia-ischemia. In addition, prolonged hypoxia-ischemia also resulted in a rapid onset of apoptosis, which occurred within 1 h after 150 min of hypoxia-ischemia, but not until 24 h after shorter hypoxic-ischemic intervals. In parallel, neuronal IGF-I expression was also affected by the duration of the hypoxia-ischemia, as observed on adjacent sections using in situ hybridization histochemistry. With hypoxia-ischemia time less than 90 min, there was no detectable change in neuronal IGF-I mRNA expression. As the hypoxia-ischemia increased to 120 min, there was a decrease in neuronal IGF-I mRNA, which was already evident within 1 h after 150 min of hypoxia-ischemia [11], whereas it had not been apparent until 24 h after 120 min of injury. By 72 h of recovery following all intervals of hypoxia-ischemia, IGF-I mRNA gene expression was activated in reactive astrocytes. This injury-induced astrocytic IGF-I expression has also been observed in other brain injury models, such as a cannula-induced lesion and focal cerebral ischemia [13, 14, 29–32]. The expression of IGF-I in reactive astrocytes is thought to be related to heightened astroglial metabolism during the 'clean-up' process following injury [11, 29, 32].

The decrease in neuronal IGF-I mRNA is not explained by dwindling metabolism during cell death because these neurons are still transcriptionally active following injury, as shown by increased expression of c-*fos*, TGFβ, nerve growth factor, c-*Jun* and two specific glucose transporters (Glut 1 and 3) [1, 20, 33]. On the other hand, IGF-I is an anabolic factor that stimulates cellular metabolism including glucose and amino acid uptake and protein synthesis [29], which is essential for cell survival. The decrease in IGF-I expression may result in a further decrease in cellular metabolism in a system already metabolically compromised. If administered within 120 min after hypoxic-ischemic injury, IGF-I prevents apoptosis in both neuronal and nonneuronal cells [18, 34, 35] and reduces neuronal loss [14, 15, 36]. IGF-I has also been shown to be a survival factor for cultured neurons isolated from stroke-prone spontaneously hypertensive rats [37, 38]. It is possible that IGF-I promotes neuronal survival following ischemic injury by regulating cellular metabolism.

Changes in IGFBP5 mRNA paralleled the changes in IGF-I mRNA. IGFBP5 gene expression is known to be temporally and spatially related to IGF-I mRNA in brain development [29] and following perinatal hypoxia-ischemia [11, 12]. IGF-I and IGFBP5 mRNA are normally coexpressed in principal neurons of sensory relay systems, with peak levels at postnatal days 12–14 [29, 39]. The coexpression of IGF-I and IGFBP5 following hypoxia-ischemia is unique to the neonatal brain and suggests a specific role for IGFBP5 in regulating the action of IGF-I in areas of injured brain at this developmental stage. Among all IGFBPs, IGFBP5 has the highest affinity for IGF-I – about 50-fold greater than that of the IGFR-I [40]. This high affinity will decrease when the IGFBP5-IGF complex binds to the extracellular matrix protein, from which IGF-I is released [41]. It is conceivable that, in the later recovery period, IGF-I and IGFBP5 are released by astrocytes in bound form, which allows diffusion to other sites in need of the anabolic action of IGF-I-I [11].

Regions of the brain respond to hypoxic-ischemic injury differently, with the cortex most sensitive and the thalamus the least. Similar regional differences in necrotic cell death following hypoxic-ischemic injury have been demonstrated; also with the most significant damage in the cortex and hippocampus, and the least in the thalamus [3, 21, 42–44]. These regional differences may occur for a variety of reasons, including differences in metabolic demand, variations in adequacy of blood flow (such as in 'watershed' areas), differences in growth factor expression, and developmental differences in the neurons and glia of the neonatal brain. Specific neuronal populations have different susceptibility to hypoxia-ischemia, reflected by the degree of apoptosis [45]. The survival of immature astrocytes during ischemia correlates with their maintenance of high-energy phosphates, with cell death occurring in those astrocytes that have a decreased ATP level below a critically 'low' threshold [46]. As an anabolic growth factor, IGF-I [12, 29], IGF-I receptor [19] and IGFBP5 [29] mRNA express at higher levels [19, 29, 39] in the thalamus than in other brain regions. This high level of IGF system gene expression is likely to contribute to the insensitivity of the thalamus to hypoxic-ischemic injury in this and one other study [12]. This proposal is supported by the fact that the greatest decrease in neuronal loss following central administration of IGF-I after hypoxia-ischemia is seen in the thalamus, amygdala, and dentate gyrus [16, 18]. Developmental changes in the neuron and glial microenvironment may also affect the ability of the neuron to respond to injury. Many cortical neurons are still migrating to their destinations in the first postnatal week [27]. Other neurons that have completed their migration differed by forming dendritic and axonal processes and synaptic connections, and producing excitatory amino acid neurotransmitters [27]. It is possible that the immature neurons are more vulnerable to hypoxic-ischemic injury shown as accelerated apoptotic cell death [8].

In conclusion, this study demonstrated that the decrease in neuronal IGF-I (and IGFBP5) after a critical hypoxic-ischemic insult correlated with an increase in the number of apoptotic cells. The critical hypoxic-ischemic insult that resulted in a decrease in neuronal IGF-I and a significant increase in apoptotic cell death occurred at approximately 120 min and intervention prior to significant apoptotic cell death narrows with more prolonged hypoxia-ischemia. Areas susceptible to less significant insult, such as the cortex, may be especially sensitive to hypoxia-ischemia induced apoptosis. In addition, the decline in neuronal IGF-I following hypoxic-ischemic injury may contribute to apoptotic cell death.

Acknowledgements

We are grateful to Mrs. Nancy Chapman for secretarial support. This study was supported by grants from the National Institutes of Health R29 NS34290 (W.-H.L.) and R29 HD31521 (S.J.V.).

References

1 Dragunow M, Beilharz E, Sirimanne E, Lawlor P, Williams C, Bravo R, Gluckman P: Immediate-early gene protein expression in neurons undergoing delayed death, but not necrosis, following hypoxic-ischaemic injury to the young rat brain. Mol Brain Res 1994;25:19–33.
2 Linnik MD, Zobrist RH, Hatfield MD: Evidence supporting a role for programmed cell death in focal cerebral ischemia in rats. Stroke 1993; 24:2002–2009.
3 Towfighi J, Yager JY, Housman C, Vannucci RC: Neuropathology of remote hypoxic-ischemic damage in the immature rat. Acta Neuropathol (Berl) 1991;81:578–587.
4 Hill IE, MacManus JP, Rasquinha I, Tuor UI: DNA fragmentation indicative of apoptosis following unilateral cerebral hypoxia-ischemia in the neonatal rat. Brain Res 1995;676: 398–403.
5 Hengartner M: Death by crowd control. Science 1998;281:1298–1299.
6 MacManus JP, Buchan AM, Hill IE, Rasquinha I, Preston E: Global ischemia can cause DNA fragmentation indicative of apoptosis in rat brain. Neurosci Lett 1993;164:89–92.
7 Mehmet H, Yue X, Squier MV, Lorek A, Cady E, Penrice J, Sarraf C, Wylezinska M, Kirkbride V, Cooper C, Brown GC, Wyatt JS, Reynolds EOR, Edwards AD: Increased apoptosis in the cingulate sulcus of newborn piglets following transient hypoxia-ischaemia is related to the degree of high energy phosphate depletion during the insult. Neurosci Lett 1994;181:121–125.
8 Yue X, Mehmet H, Penrice J, Cooper C, Cady E, Wyatt JS, Raynolds EOR, Edwards AD, Squier MV: Apoptosis and necrosis in the newborn piglet brain following transient cerebral hypoxia-ischaemia. Neuropathol Appl Neurobiol 1997;23:16–25.
9 Bursch W, Kleine L, Tenniswood M: The biochemistry of cell death by apoptosis. Biochem Cell Biol 1990; 68:1071–1074.
10 Guenettte RS, Tenniswood M: The role of growth factors in the suppression of active cell death in the prostate: An hypothesis. Biochem Cell Biol 1994;72:553–559.
11 Lee W-H, Wang G-M, Seaman LB, Vannucci SJ: Coordinate IGF-I and IGFBP5 gene expression in perinatal rat brain after hypoxia-ischemia. J Cereb Blood Flow Metab 1996;16: 227–236.
12 Beilharz EJ, Klempt ND, Klempt M, Sirimanne E, Dragunow M, Gluckman PD: Differential expression of insulin-like growth factor binding proteins (IGFBP) 4 and 5 mRNA in the rat brain after transient hypoxic-ischemic injury. Mol Brain Res 1993;18:209–215.
13 Garcia-Estrada J, Garcia-Segura LM, Torres-Aleman I: Expression of insulin-like growth factor I by astrocytes in response to injury. Brain Res 1992;592:343–347.
14 Gluckman P, Klempt N, Guan J, Mallard C, Sirimanne E, Dragunow M, Klempt M, Singh K, Williams C, Nikolics K: A role for IGF-1 in the rescue of CNS neurons following hypoxic-ischemic injury. Biochem Biophys Res Commun 1992;182: 593–599.
15 Gluckman PD, Guan J, Williams CE, Johnston BM, Beilharz E: Insulin-like growth factors (IGFs) in the injured central nervous system. Abstr Soc Endo 1994;76:2D:3.
16 Guan J, Williams C, Gunning M, Mallard C, Gluckman P: The effects of IGF-1 treatment after hypoxic-ischemic brain injury in adult rats. J Cereb Blood Flow Metab 1993;13: 609–616.
17 Johnson NL, Gardner AM, Diener KM, Lange-Carter CA, Gleavy J, Jarpe MB, Minden A, Karin M, Zon LI, Johnson GL: Signal transduction pathways regulated by mitogen-activated extracellular response kinase kinase kinase induce cell death. J Biol Chem 1996;271:3229–3237.
18 Johnston BM, Mallard EC, Williams CE, Gluckman PD: Insulin-like growth factor-1 is a potent neuronal rescue agent after hypoxic-ischemic injury in fetal lambs. J Clin Invest 1996;97:300–308.
19 Bondy CA, Bach MA, Lee W-H: Mapping of brain insulin and insulin-like growth factor receptor gene expression by in situ hybridization. Neuroprotocols 1992;1:240–249.
20 Klempt ND, Klempt M, Gunn AJ, Singh K, Gluckman PD: Expression of insulin-like growth factor-binding protein 2 (IGF-BP 2) following transient hypoxia-ischemia in the infant rat brain. Mol Brain Res 1992;15: 55–61.
21 Rice JE III, Vannucci RC, Brierley JB: The influence of immaturity on hypoxic-ischemic brain damage in the rat. Ann Neurol 1981;9:131–141.
22 Gavrieli Y, Sherman Y, Ben-Sasson SA: Identification of programmed cell death in situ via specific labeling of nuclear DNA fragmentation. J Cell Biol 1992;119:493–501.
23 Zhou J, Bondy CA: Anatomy of the human ovarian IGF system. Biol Reprod 1993;48:467–482.
24 Modak SP, Bollum FJ: Terminal lens cell differentiation. III. Initiator activity of DNA during nuclear degeneration. Exp Cell Res 1970;62: 421–432.
25 Ferrer I, Macaya A, Blanco R, Olivé M, Cinós C, Munell F, Planas AM: Evidence of internucleosomal DNA fragmentation and identification of dying cells in X-ray-induced cell death in the developing brain. Intl J Devel Neurosci 1995;13:21–28.
26 Linnik MD, Miller JA, Sprinkle-Cavallo J, Mason PJ, Thompson FY, Montgomery LR, Schroeder KK: Apoptotic DNA fragmentation in the rat cerebral cortex induced by permanent middle cerebral artery occlusion. Mol Brain Res 1995;32: 116–124.
27 Grafe MR: Developmental changes in the sensitivity of the neonatal rat brain to hypoxic/ischemic injury. Brain Res 1994;653:161–166.
28 Hepler JE, Lund PK: Molecular biology of the insulin-like growth factors: Relevance to nervous system function. Mol Neurobiol 1990;4:93–127.

29 Bondy CA, Lee W-H: Patterns of insulin-like growth factor and IGF receptor gene expression in the brain. Ann NY Acad Sci 1993;692: 33–43
30 Clemmons DR: IGF binding proteins: Regulation of cellular actions. Growth Regul 1992;2:80–87.
31 Guan J, Skinner SJM, Beilharz EJ, Hua KM, Hodgkinson S, Gluckman PD, Williams CE: Movement of IGF-I into the brain parenchyma after hypoxic-ischaemic injury. Neuroreport 1996;7:632–636.
32 Lee W-H, Clemens JA, Bondy CA: Insulin-like growth factors in the response to cerebral ischemia. Mol Cell Neurosci 1992;3:36–43.
33 Lee W-H, Bondy CA: Ischemic injury induces brain glucose transporter gene expression. Endocrinology 1993;133:2540–2544.
34 Neff NT, Prevette D, Houenou LJ, Lewis ME, Glicksman MA, Yin Q-W, Oppenheim RW: Insulin-like growth factors: Putative muscle-derived trophic agents that promote motoneuron survival. J Neurobiol 1993;24:1578–1588.
35 Rodriguez-Tarduchy G, Collins MKL, García I, López-Rivas A: Insulin-like growth factor-I inhibits apoptosis in il-3-dependent hemopoietic cells. J Immunol 1992;149: 535–540.
36 Guan J, Williams CE, Skinner SJM, Mallard EC, Gluckman PD: The effects of insulin-like growth factor (IGF)-1, IGF-2, and des-IGF-1 on neuronal loss after hypoxic-ischemic brain injury in adult rats: Evidence for a role for IGF binding proteins. Endocrinology 1996;137:893–898.
37 Tagami M, Yamagata K, Nara Y, Fujino H, Kubota A, Numano F, Yamori Y: Insulin-like growth factors prevent apoptosis in cortical neurons isolated from stroke-prone spontaneously hypertensive rats. Lab Invest 1997;76:603–612.
38 Tagami M, Ikeda K, Nara Y, Fujino H, Kubota A, Numano F, Yamori Y: Insulin-like growth factor-1 attenuates apoptosis in hippocampal neurons caused by cerebral ischemia and reperfusion in stroke-prone spontaneously hypertensive rats. Lab Invest 1997;76:613–617.
39 Bondy CA: Transient IGF-I gene expression during the maturation of functionally related central projection neurons. J Neurosci 1991;11: 3442–3455.
40 Cohick WS, Clemmons DR: The insulin-like growth factors. Annu Rev Physiol 1993;55:131–153.
41 Jones JI, Gockerman A, Busby WH Jr, Camacho-Hubner C, Clemmons DR: Extracellular matrix contains insulin-like growth factor binding protein-5: Potentiation of the effects of IGF-I. J Cell Biol 1993;121:679–687.
42 Pulsinelli WA, Brierley JB, Plum F: Temporal profile of neuronal damage in a model of transient forebrain ischemia. Ann Neurol 1982;11:491–498.
43 Tuor UI, Del Bigio MR, Chumas PD: Brain damage due to cerebral hypoxia/ischemia in the neonate. Cerebrovasc Brain Metab Rev 1996; 8:159–193.
44 Williams CE, Gunn AJ, Mallard C, Gluckman PD: Outcome after ischemia in the developing sheep brain: An electroencephalographic and histological study. Ann Neurol 1992; 31:14–21.
45 Charriaut-Marlangue C, Margaill I, Represa A, Popovici T, Plotkine M, Ben-Ari Y: Apoptosis and necrosis after reversible focal ischemia: An in situ DNA fragmentation analysis. J Cereb Blood Flow Metab 1996;16: 186–194.
46 Yager JY, Kala G, Hertz L, Juurlink BHJ: Correlation between content of high-energy phosphates and hypoxic-ischemic damage in immature and mature astrocytes. Dev Brain Res 1994;82:62–68.

Biological Signals and Receptors

Biol Signals Recept 1999;8:294–308

Received: November 13, 1998
Accepted: February 12, 1999

Neurophysiological Changes Associated with Selective Neuronal Damage in Hippocampus following Transient Forebrain Ischemia

Zao C. Xu[a] Tian-Ming Gao[b] Yubo Ren[c]

[a]Department of Anatomy, Indiana University School of Medicine, Indianapolis, Ind., USA;
[b]Department of Physiology, The First Military Medical University, Guangzhou, China, and
[c]Department of Neuroscience, Ottawa Civic Hospital, Ottawa, Ont., Canada

Key Words

Ischemia · Hippocampus · Excitotoxicity · Synaptic potentiation · Synaptic depression · In vivo intracellular recording

Abstract

Neurophysiological changes of hippocampal neurons were compared before and after transient forebrain ischemia using intracellular recording and staining techniques in vivo. Ischemic depolarization (ID) was used as an indication of severe ischemia. Under halothane anesthesia, approximately 13 min of ID consistently produced severe neuronal damage in the CA1 region of rat hippocampus, while CA3 pyramidal neurons and dentate granule cells remained intact. After such severe ischemia, approximately 60% of the CA1 neurons exhibited a synaptic potentiation. The excitability of these neurons progressively decreased following reperfusion. Approximately 30% of the CA1 neurons showed a synaptic depression following ischemia. The excitability of these neurons transiently decreased following reperfusion. After ischemia of the same severity, both synaptic transmission and excitability of CA3 and granule cells transiently depressed. These data suggest that ischemia-induced synaptic potentiation may be associated with the pathogenesis of neuronal damage following ischemia, and that the synaptic depression may have protective effects on hippocampal neurons after ischemic insult.

KARGER

Fax +41 61 306 12 34
E-Mail karger@karger.ch
www.karger.com

Accessible online at:
http://BioMedNet.com/karger

Zao C. Xu, MD, PhD, Department of Anatomy, MS507
Indiana University School of Medicine
635 Barnhill Drive, Indianapolis, IN 46202 (USA)
Tel. +1 317 274 0547, Fax +1 317 278 2040
E-Mail zxu@anatomy.iupui.edu

Introduction

The neurons in the central nervous system are highly sensitive to cerebral ischemia. Vulnerability to ischemia varies widely among different regions in the brain [1, 2]. Different neuronal populations within a brain region also show different susceptibilities to ischemic insult. Studies have shown that CA1 pyramidal neurons in the hippocampus die 3–7 days after transient forebrain ischemia, while CA3 neurons and dentate granule cells in the same region remain intact [3, 4]. The mechanisms of this selective neuronal damage are not fully understood. Excessive accumulation of extracellular glutamate during ischemia has been postulated to cause neuronal hyperactivity and excessive Ca^{2+} influx; intracellular free Ca^{2+} then triggers the process of neuronal injury [5, 6]. However, the electrophysiological evidence for hyperactivity in the hippocampus after ischemia remains a controversial issue. Using extracellular recording techniques in vivo, some studies showed an increase [7, 8], while others showed a decrease [9–11] in neuronal firing rate in the CA1 area following ischemia. In addition to spontaneous firing, the electrophysiological properties and synaptic transmission following brief cerebral ischemia may participate in the pathophysiological mechanisms that cause selective neuronal damage. Using intracellular recording techniques in vitro, several studies indicated that neuronal activity and synaptic transmission are suppressed during hypoxia and after reoxygenation [12–14]. However, data from in vitro studies should be interpreted cautiously with respect to their relevance to in vivo ischemia. Besides the traumatic process of preparing the brain slices, the temperature, composition of the interstitial fluid, and oxygen and glucose levels in vitro dramatically differ from those in vivo. Each of these variables alone crucially affects the outcome of ischemia, as well as the neurophysiological responses of the neuron. In an attempt to circumvent such problems with anoxia in brain slices, some investigators induced ischemia in vivo and then prepared brain slices for recording at different time points following reperfusion. Using this approach, some studies showed enhanced excitatory transmission shortly after reperfusion [15–18], but other studies showed no evidence of hyperactivity [19] or decreased excitability of CA1 neurons [18]. In contrast to the above approaches, in vivo intracellular recordings preserve the complex system physiology while permitting the detection of changes in neuronal and synaptic activities.

In order to identify the electrophysiological changes associated with mechanisms of postischemic cell death in the hippocampus, the present study examined the spontaneous firing, evoked synaptic potentials and excitability of ischemia-vulnerable neurons (CA1 pyramidal neurons) and ischemia-resistant neurons (CA3 pyramidal neurons, dentate granule cells), following severe forebrain ischemia using intracellular recording and staining techniques in vivo.

Methods

Transient Forebrain Ischemia

Male adult Wistar rats (250–350 g, Charles River) were subjected to transient forebrain ischemia using the 4-vessel occlusion method (4-VO) [20] with modifications. The animals were fasted overnight to provide uniform blood glucose levels. For surgical preparation, the animals were anesthetized with 1–2% halothane mixed with 33% O_2 and 66% N_2. An occluding device (a loop of silicone tubing) was placed loosely around each carotid artery. The caudal artery was cannulated for monitoring of the arterial blood pressure (BP) and taking blood samples for blood gas tension analysis. The arterial P_{O_2} was maintained at approximately 120 mm Hg, and the P_{CO_2} at <40 mm Hg. The animal was then placed on a stereotaxic frame, and the core body temperature was maintained at 37°C

Table 1. Physiological parameters and arterial gas tension during experiments

	BP mm Hg	pH	Pa_{CO_2} mm Hg	Pa_{O_2} mm Hg	Hb %	Glucose mg/dl
Mean	87.0	7.33	37.2	123.0	43	84
SD	5.6	0.04	4.0	14.7	4	14
n	57	57	56	56	57	57

BP = Blood pressure; Hb = hemoglobin.

through a temperature control unit (TC-120, Medical System). The vertebral arteries were electrocauterized. A small temperature probe (0.8 mm OD) was inserted beneath the skull in the extradural space after which brain temperature was maintained at 37 °C with a heating lamp. Severe forebrain ischemia was induced by occluding both common carotid arteries to induce ischemic depolarization for approximately 14 min.

Recording of Ischemic Depolarization

The extracellular direct current (DC) potential in the CA1 region of the hippocampus was monitored during ischemia. Recording microelectrodes were pulled from glass capillaries (A-M system) to a tip resistance of approximately 5 MΩ when filled with 2 *M* NaCl. A burr hole was drilled at 4.0 mm anterior to the interaural line and 3.0 mm from the midline. A microelectrode was inserted into the CA1 region (~2.5 mm below the brain surface). Following baseline recordings, forebrain ischemia was initiated by tightening the occluding device. The DC potential, cerebral blood flow (CBF) and arterial BP were digitized with the data acquisition program Superscope (GW Instrument).

Intracellular Recording and Staining

The animals were anesthetized with 1–2% halothane. The skull was opened to expose the cortex above the recording site and for placement of stimulus electrodes. To evoke synaptic responses from CA1 neurons, a pair of bipolar stimulating electrodes was placed in the contralateral commissural pathway (anteroposterior (AP) 3.7–4.7, mediolateral (ML) 1.5, and dorsoventral (DV) 3.5 mm, interaural), and used to deliver constant current pulses of 0.1 ms duration. For CA3 and granule cells, the stimulating electrode was placed into the ipsilateral perforant pathway at a 25° angle to the vertical (AP 1.5, ML 1.5–2.5, and DV 4.0 mm). Recording electrodes were pulled from glass capillaries with filaments (A-M System) to a tip resistance of 40–70 MΩ when filled with a solution of 3% neurobiotin (Vector) in 2 *M* potassium acetate. Cerebral spinal fluid was drained via a cisternal puncture, and the animals were suspended by a clamp applied to their tails. After placement of a microelectrode in the cortex above the hippocampus for recording, the exposed surface of the brain was covered with soft paraffin wax.

Neurons with stable membrane potentials were selected for study. Data were digitized with Axodata (Axon Instrument) and stored for off-line analysis. After each successful recording, neurobiotin was iontophoresed into the cell by passing depolarizing current pulses (2 Hz, 300 ms, 1–1.5 nA) for 15–30 min. At the end of the experiment, the animal was perfused transcardially with 4% paraformaldehyde. The brain was removed and stored in fixative overnight. Coronal vibratome sections were cut at 50-μm thickness, and incubated in 0.1% peroxidase-conjugated avidin-D (Vector) in 0.01 *M* potassium-phosphate-buffered saline (KPBS) with 0.5% Triton X-100 overnight at room temperature for 6–8 h. After detection of peroxidase activity with 3′,3′-diaminobenzidine, sections were examined in KPBS. Sections containing intracellularly stained neurons were mounted on gelatin-coated slides and processed for histological observation.

Results

Temporal Threshold of Maximal CA1 Cell Damage

In the present study, forebrain ischemia was induced under halothane anesthesia, and the brain temperature of the animals was maintained at 37 °C, which was different from the original 4-VO model. Therefore, ex-

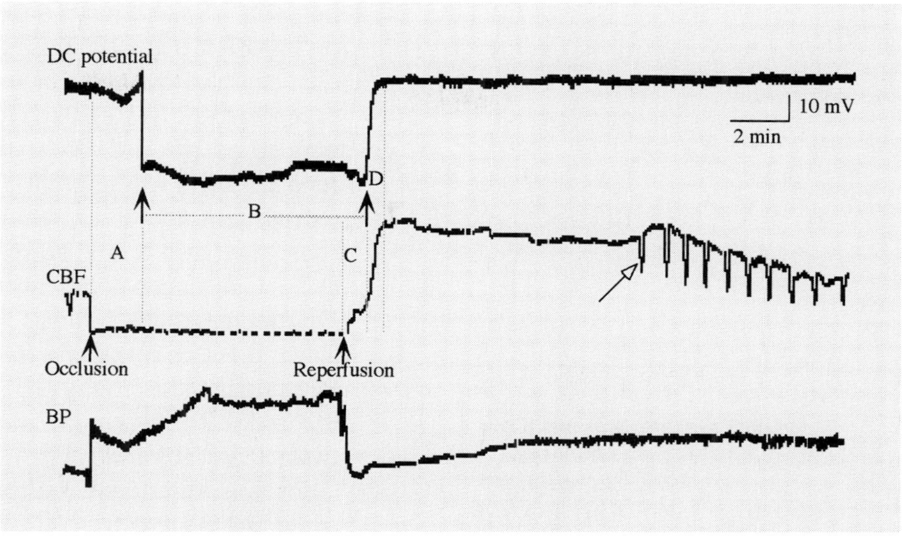

Fig. 1. Example of DC potential, CBF and BP before, during and shortly after ischemia. The upper recording shows the DC potential, where the arrows indicate the beginning and end of ID. The middle recording shows the blood flow monitored from the cerebral cortex, where the filled arrows indicate the beginning of occlusion and reperfusion, respectively, and the open arrow indicates the interruption caused by illumination of the heating lamp. The lower recording shows the BP measured through the caudal artery. A represents the period of DL; B represents the ID time; C represents the RD time, and D represents the RT. Immediately after 4-VO, CBF dropped to <10% of control levels and BP increased. Approximately 1.7 min after occlusion, the DC potential quickly hyperpolarized to about –24 mV and remained at this level throughout ischemia. After reperfusion, BP was immediately reduced. CBF gradually returned to preischemic levels and then increased dramatically. This hyperperfusion lasted about 30 min, and then gradually returned to the preischemic level. The DC potential remained at –24 mV for about 1 min, and then repolarized to the preischemic level.

periments were conducted to determine the temporal threshold of maximal postischemic damage in the CA1 region under our experimental conditions. The arterial gas tension and general physiological parameters of these animals were maintained in normal ranges (table 1). Immediately after occlusion of the common carotid arteries, CBF was reduced to <10% of the preischemic level and BP was increased. The DC potential remained unchanged for about 2 min and then quickly hyperpolarized to approximately –20 mV and stayed at this level throughout ischemia. After reperfusion, BP dropped immediately, while CBF gradually returned to the preischemic level and then increased dramatically (postischemic hyperperfusion). After releasing, DC potential was maintained at –20 mV for approximately 1 min before quickly returning to the preischemic level. Figure 1 shows an example of changes in DC potential, CBF and BP during experiments. The DC potential changes of groups 1–4 during the experiments were measured and shown in table 2. As illustrated in figure 1, depolarization latency (DL) is the time between the occlusion of common carotid arteries and the start of ischemic depolarization (ID). ID is the time that the DC

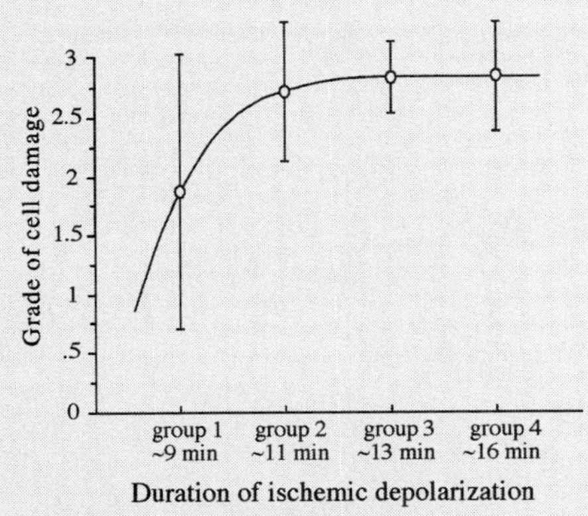

CA1 cell damage following ischemia

Group	N	Mean	SD
1	16	1.88	1.16
2	20	2.73*	0.60
3	16	2.84*	0.30
4	20	2.85**	0.46

N is the number of hemispheres. ** P<0.01; * P<0.05 compared with group 1 using nonparametric Mann-Whitney U test.

Fig. 2. Relationship between ID and CA1 cell damage. The values are means, and error bars are SD of groups 1–4. If ID was reduced to 9 min, cell damage decreased to 1.88 ± 1.16. According to the curve, the temporal threshold for maximal CA1 cell damage following ischemia is at about 12 min ID.

potential is maintained at about –20 mV. Repolarization delay (RD) is the time between the release of the occlusion and the beginning of repolarization. Repolarization time (RT) is defined as the time from the beginning of repolarization to the point at which DC potentials return to their preischemic levels. Because the brain temperature was maintained at 37 °C during experiments, the variation of DL among groups 1–4 was very small, being 2.1 ± 0.5–2.5 ± 0.8 min (mean ± SD). The RD among these groups varied between 0.9 ± 0.2 and 1.7 ± 1.1 min, and RT varied between 0.8 ± 0.3 and 1.5 ± 1.1 min. No correlation was found between the length of ischemia and the length of RD and RT. Because of the relatively small variation in DL and RD, the ID is approximately 1 min shorter than the time of occlusion in each group.

In order to examine the postischemic damage, the animals were sacrificed 7 days after ischemia. Coronal vibratome sections (50 μm) were cut and stained with hematoxylin and eosin. The sections were examined with a light microscope, and neuronal damage was graded on a scale of 0 to 3 with 0 = normal brain; 1 = a few neurons damaged; 2 = many neurons damaged, and 3 = the majority of neurons damaged [4]. The relationship be-

Table 2. Electrophysiological parameters during experiments

Group	n	Depolarization latency, min	Ischemic depolarization, min	Repolarization delay, min	Repolarization time, min
1	8	2.1 ± 0.5	8.7 ± 0.6	0.9 ± 0.2	1.4 ± 0.4
2	10	2.5 ± 0.8	11.5 ± 1.0	1.4 ± 1.1	1.2 ± 0.6
3	8	2.4 ± 0.6	13.0 ± 0.3	1.1 ± 0.3	0.9 ± 0.2
4	10	2.3 ± 1.1	16.0 ± 1.0	0.8 ± 1.0	1.4 ± 1.1

The values are means ± SD.

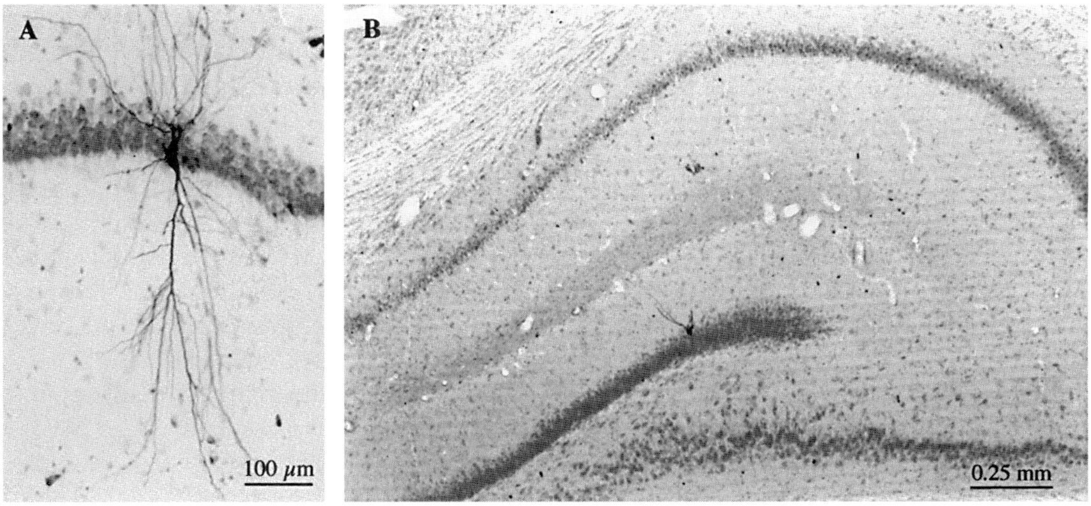

Fig. 3. Photomicrographs of intracellularly stained neurons after ischemia. **A** Example of CA1 neurons recorded 8 h after reperfusion. **B** A coronal section of hippocampus 48 h after reperfusion. The section was counterstained with hematoxylin and eosin. Neurons in the medial portion of the CA1 region have degenerated and a dentate granule cell was intracellularly stained.

tween ID duration and extent of cell damage is illustrated in figure 2. The data indicate that if ID duration is <11 min, the extent of CA1-cell damage decreases and the variation increases dramatically. At approximately 12 min of ID, the extent of cell damage begins to level off, suggesting that maximal cell damage has been reached. Therefore, ischemia that induced an ID of approximately 13 min was adapted in the present study as a criterion of severe forebrain ischemia.

Electrophysiological Changes in CA1 Neurons after Ischemia

Intracellular recording and staining in vivo were performed before and up to 2 days after severe forebrain ischemia. The recorded neurons were identified as CA1 neurons by intracellular staining, as shown in figure 3A. In control animals, stimulation of the contralateral commissural pathway (CC) elicited excitatory postsynaptic potentials (EPSPs) from CA1 pyramidal neurons, followed by inhibitory potentials (IPSPs) (fig. 4A). The same stimuli elicited three different responses from CA1 pyramidal neurons after ischemia. Approximately 60% of the neurons exhibited a late depolarizing postsynaptic potential (L-PSP) in addition to the initial EPSP (fig. 4B). The L-PSPs were elicited as early as 4 h and as late as 48 h after reperfusion. More than 30% of the neurons failed to develop L-PSPs upon CC stimulation and exhibited moderately attenuated synaptic responses (fig. 4C). A smaller group of neurons (~10%) also failed to develop L-PSPs, but the synaptic responses of these neurons were more severely attenuated (fig. 4D). These three groups were designated as L-PSP, non-L-PSP and small excitatory postsynaptic potential (S-EPSP) neurons, respectively.

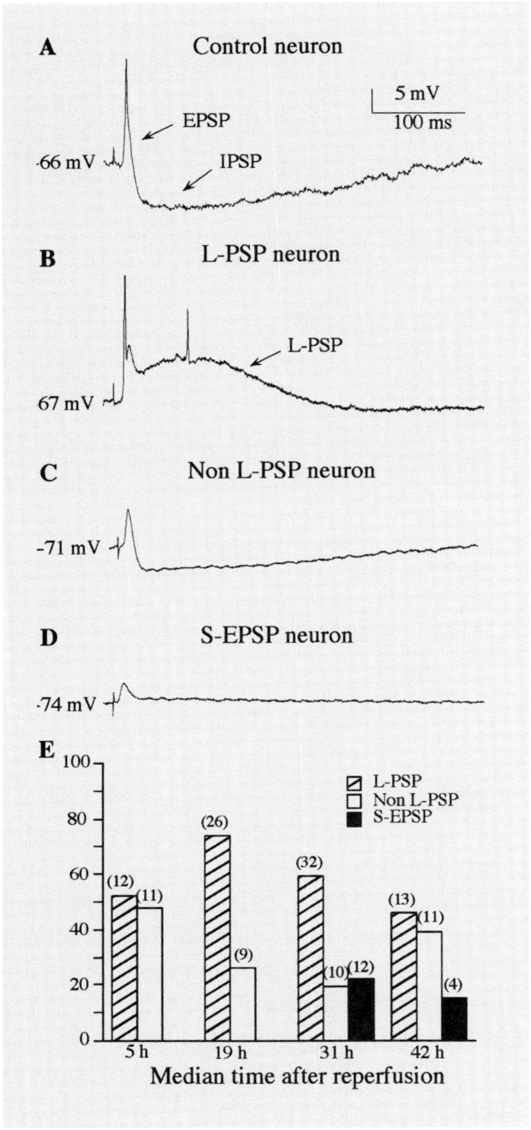

Fig. 4. Evoked synaptic responses from CA1 neurons before and after transient forebrain ischemia. **A** Recording from a control rat in which stimulation of the contralateral CC elicited an EPSP followed by an IPSP. An action potential was triggered by the EPSP. **B** After ischemia, the same stimulus evoked an additional L-PSP from approximately 60% of the CA1 neurons. Action potentials were occasionally triggered by L-PSPs. **C** In approximately 30% of the neurons, CC stimuli elicited an EPSP/IPSP sequence with a smaller amplitude in comparison with control neurons. **D** Approximately 31 h after reperfusion, a small EPSP was evoked from approximately 10% of the neurons even with maximal stimulus intensity. Traces in **B–D** were recorded 27, 35 and 28 h after reperfusion, respectively. Each trace is the average of 4 recordings. The action potentials in these figures are truncated. The scales in **A** also apply to **B–D**. **E** Proportions of 3 distinct responses in CA1 neurons at different periods following reperfusion. The percentage of L-PSP neurons gradually increased and peaked at approximately 19 h, while the percentage of non-L-PSP neurons progressively decreased following reperfusion. The number of recorded neurons is in parentheses.

In order to study the dynamics of electrophysiological responses after reperfusion, the neurons were pooled according to the reperfusion time during which they were recorded: 0–12 h (median 5 h); 13–24 h (median 19 h); 25–36 h (median 31 h), and 37–48 h (median 42 h). The number of L-PSP and non-L-PSP neurons was approximately equal during the first 12 h of reperfusion (fig. 4E). The proportion of L-PSP neurons increased to >70% during 13–24 h and declined slightly thereafter, while S-EPSP neurons composed approximately 20% of the population after 24 h. In contrast, the percentage of non-L-PSP neurons progressively decreased through 36 h. It should be noted that during 37–48 h after reperfusion, it was difficult to record from the medial portion of the CA1 zone because most neurons in this region had degenerated (fig. 3B).

The characteristics of PSPs evoked by CC stimulation at 2.5 times the threshold stimulus intensity were compared before ischemia and at intervals after reperfusion. The slope of initial EPSPs in L-PSP neurons increased to 155% of control neurons ($p < 0.05$, ANOVA) around 5 h after reperfusion (fig. 5A), suggesting that a synaptic facilitation was induced in these neurons by transient ischemia. The

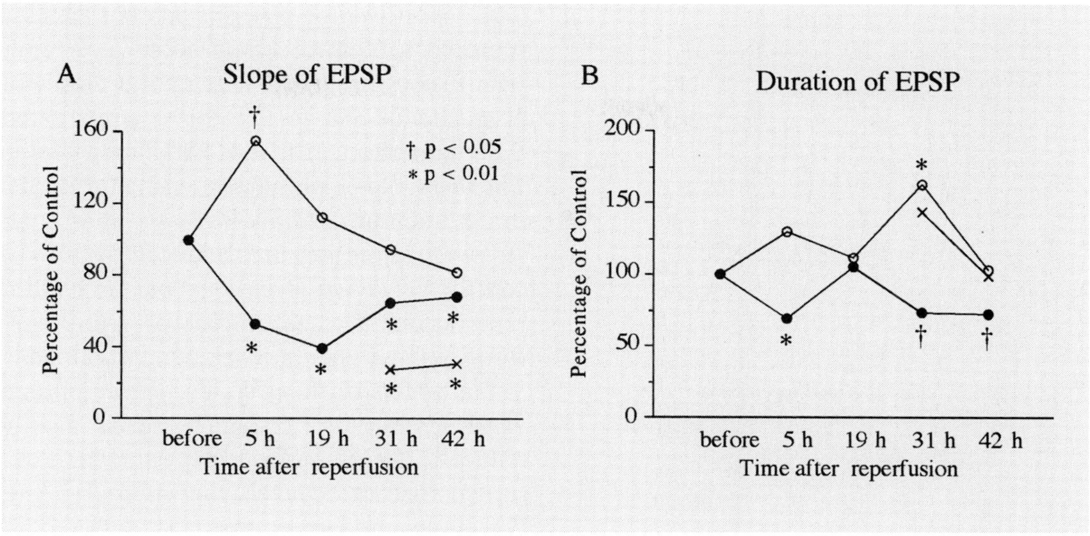

Fig. 5. Plots of the changes of initial EPSPs evoked from CA1 neurons by CC stimulation after ischemia. Each point is the mean value of percentage as compared with that before ischemia. **A** The slope of initial EPSPs of neurons with L-PSPs was significantly enhanced around 5 h after reperfusion ($p < 0.05$, ANOVA), and gradually returned to preischemic levels approximately 31 h after reperfusion. In non-L-PSP neurons, however, the slope was persistently lower than preischemic values up to approximately 42 h following reperfusion ($p < 0.01$). A remarkable reduction in the slope of initial EPSPs was also observed in S-EPSP neurons ($p < 0.01$). **B** The duration of the initial EPSP in L-PSP neurons gradually increased, while that of non-L-PSP neurons decreased.

slope of initial EPSPs returned to the preischemic level 19 h after reperfusion. In contrast, the slope of initial EPSPs in non-L-PSP neurons progressively decreased to as low as 40% of control levels around 19 h after reperfusion ($p < 0.01$), suggesting that ischemia induced a synaptic depression in this subgroup of CA1 neurons. The slope of initial EPSPs in S-EPSP neurons was dramatically depressed at all times ($p < 0.01$). The changes in slope were consistent with the changes in amplitude of initial EPSPs in all three neuron types (data not shown). The duration of initial EPSPs was progressively longer in L-PSP neurons and shorter in non-L-PSP neurons than observed in control neurons (fig. 5B). Spontaneous firing in CA1 neurons ceased shortly after ischemia and never returned to control levels up to 48 h following reperfusion.

The changes in neuronal excitability were evaluated by comparing the spike threshold and rheobase of CA1 neurons before and after ischemia. The spike threshold was measured at the beginning of the upstroke of the first action potential, and the rheobase was determined as the minimal intensity of depolarizing current pulse to trigger an action potential. As shown in figure 6, the spike threshold and rheobase of L-PSP and S-EPSP neurons progressively increased after reperfusion, while only a transient increase in spike threshold ($p < 0.05$, ANOVA) and rheobase ($p < 0.01$, ANOVA) was detected in non-L-PSP neurons at 5 h after reperfusion.

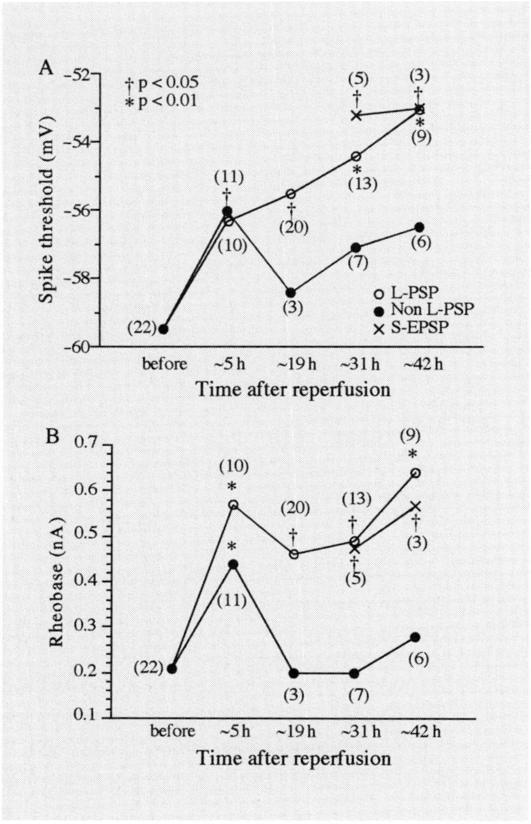

Fig. 6. Plotting of the changes in spike threshold (**A**) and rheobase (**B**) of CA1 pyramidal neurons at different intervals after reperfusion. The value of each plot is the mean, with the number of neurons in parentheses. The spike threshold and rheobase of L-PSP and S-EPSP neurons gradually increased following reperfusion, indicating a progressive decrease of neuronal excitability. However, a transient increase in spike threshold and rheobase was observed in non-L-PSP neurons in the early reperfusion period.

Electrophysiological Changes in CA3 and Granule Cells after Ischemia

The postsynaptic potentials were evoked from CA3 and granule cells by stimulation of the ipsilateral perforant pathway at 2.5 times the threshold stimulus intensity. In CA3 neurons, the amplitude of EPSPs decreased to approximately 50% of control values ($p < 0.01$) shortly after reperfusion, but quickly returned to control levels about 21 h after reperfusion (fig. 7E). The temporal profile of postischemic changes in EPSP slope exhibited a similar pattern as that of EPSP amplitudes. The threshold of stimulus intensity for EPSPs in CA3 neurons slightly increased shortly after reperfusion and then reduced to 50% of control values ($p < 0.05$) about 21 h after reperfusion. The threshold for EPSPs returned to preischemic levels at approximately 29 h after reperfusion (fig. 7F). The amplitude of EPSPs evoked from granule cells slightly reduced 19–31 h after reperfusion and returned to control levels thereafter (fig. 8E). No statistical significance was detected in these changes. Similar changes in the rising slope of EPSPs were observed in granule cells after reperfusion. The stimulus intensity threshold for EPSPs in granule cells increased shortly after reperfusion and then returned to control values around 19 h after reperfusion (fig. 8F). No statistical significance was detected in these changes.

After reperfusion, the spike threshold of CA3 and granule cells was unchanged within the first 24 h, but significantly increased at approximately 30 h ($p < 0.05$) and then returned to control values (fig. 9A, C), indicating a transient decrease in neuronal excitability after ischemia. The rheobase of CA3 neurons slightly fluctuated after reperfusion, but was not significantly different from the preischemic values (fig. 9B). The rheobase of granule cells, however, increased from 0.28 ± 0.16 nA before ischemia to 0.57 ± 0.36 nA around 31 h after reperfusion ($p < 0.01$), and then gradually returned to 0.34 ± 0.21 nA 7 days after reperfusion (fig. 9D). The spontaneous firing rate in CA3 and granule cells following ischemia remained about the same as that in control neurons.

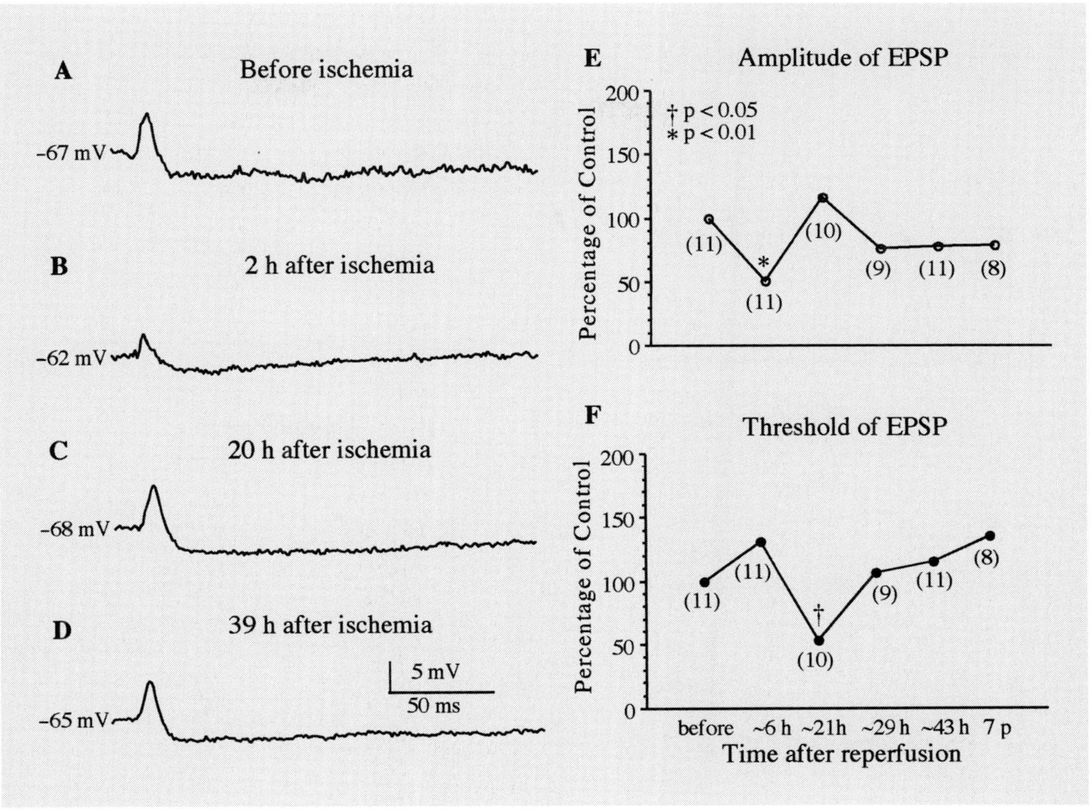

Fig. 7. Evoked PSPs of CA3 neurons before and after ischemia. **A–D** Examples of evoked PSPs elicited by the stimulation of ipsilateral perforant paths at different intervals after reperfusion. All traces are the average of 4 recordings. The scales in **D** apply to all traces. **E** Plots of temporal changes in the amplitude of EPSPs following reperfusion. The amplitude of EPSPs significantly decreased to 50% of the control value shortly after reperfusion, and then returned to preischemic levels at 21 h after reperfusion. Each point is the mean value of percentage as compared with that before ischemia. The number of neurons in each group is in parentheses. **F** Plots of the changes in the stimulus intensity threshold for inducing EPSPs. A transient decrease in stimulus threshold occurred at approximately 21 h after reperfusion.

Discussion

The present study demonstrates that severe ischemia in vivo induces two distinct changes of synaptic transmission in CA1 pyramidal neurons. Synaptic transmission in the majority of the neurons was facilitated, as evidenced by L-PSPs and enhancement of initial EPSP. The excitability of L-PSP neurons progressively decreased following reperfusion. In contrast, synaptic transmission in a subpopulation of CA1 neurons was suppressed, as evidenced by synaptic depression after ischemia. The excitability of non-L-PSP neurons transiently decreased after ischemia. On the other hand, the synaptic transmission and excitability of CA3 and granule cells transiently depressed following severe ischemic insult.

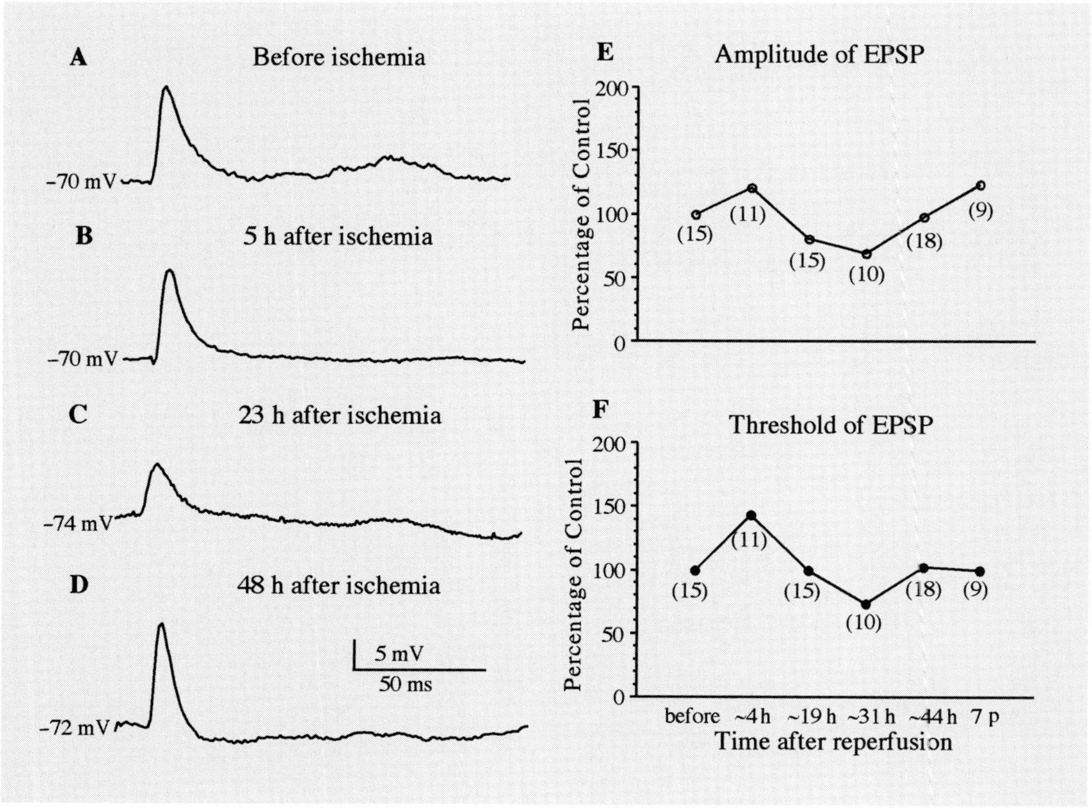

Fig. 8. Postsynaptic potentials evoked from granule cells by the stimulation of ipsilateral perforant paths before and after ischemia. **A–D** Representative recordings of EPSP amplitudes at different intervals after reperfusion. All traces are the average of 4 recordings. Scales in **D** apply to all traces. **E** Plots of changes in EPSP amplitudes following reperfusion. Each point is the mean value of percentage as compared with that before ischemia. The number of neurons in each group is in parentheses. A slight decrease in amplitude was observed during 19–31 h after reperfusion, and then returned to control values. **F** Plots of the changes in stimulus intensity threshold for inducing EPSPs in granule cells. No significant change in stimulus intensity thresholds to evoke EPSPs was found after reperfusion.

These data suggest that the enhancement of synaptic transmission and decrease of excitability may play an important role in the pathophysiological of neuronal injury following transient forebrain ischemia. The depression of synaptic transmission may have protective effects on hippocampal neurons after ischemic insult.

Facilitation and Depression of Synaptic Transmission in CA1 Neurons after Ischemia

The ischemia-induced synaptic facilitation includes two components: The increase in amplitude and slope of initial EPSPs and the development of L-PSPs. The synaptic facilitation observed in the present study resembles anoxic long-term potentiation (LTP) induced in CA1 neurons in vitro [21]. Anoxic LTP is

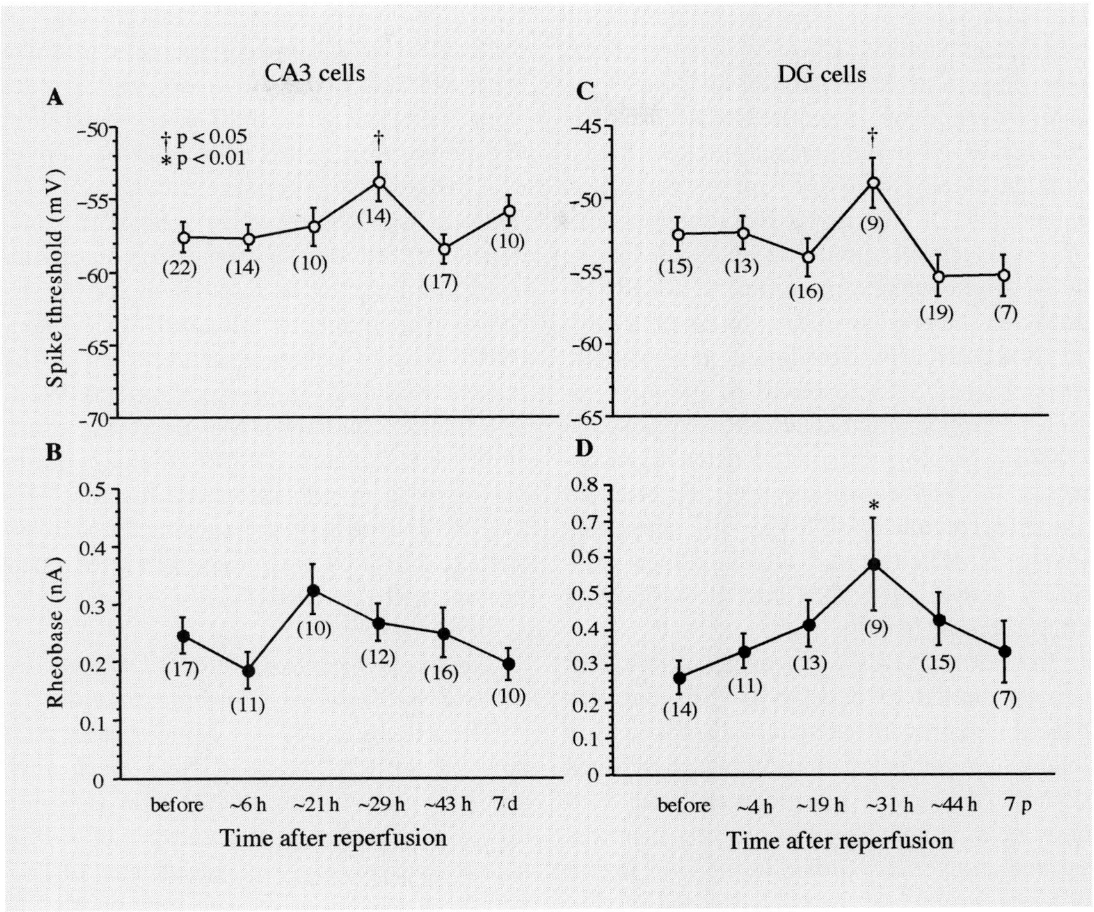

Fig. 9. Plotting of the changes in spike threshold and rheobase of CA3 neurons (**A, B**) and granule cells (**C, D**) at different periods after reperfusion. The value of each plot is the mean, with the number of neurons in parentheses. The spike threshold of both CA3 and granule cells transiently increased approximately 30 h following reperfusion, indicating a transient decrease of neuronal excitability. No significant change in rheobase was observed in CA3 neurons. A significant increase in rheobase was found at approximately 31 h after reperfusion.

selectively mediated by NMDA receptors and requires a rise in intracellular Ca^{2+} [22]. It is likely that the increase of glutamate concentration during ischemia combined with membrane potential depolarization during ID [23, 24] induces Ca^{2+} influx via ligand- and voltage-regulated Ca^{2+} channels. Elevated intracellular Ca^{2+} may then trigger Ca^{2+}-dependent facilitation of synaptic activity via phosphorylation of NMDA and AMPA receptors [25–27]. These in turn may be responsible for the long-lasting changes in synaptic efficacy observed in this study. Previous studies have shown that CA1 pyramidal neurons in hippocampal slices prepared 28 h after ischemia exhibited prolonged synaptic responses, the later components of which were blocked by NMDA antagonists [15]. In vivo extracellular recordings also demonstrated an NMDA-receptor-dependent potentiation at Schaffer collateral/CA1 pyramidal cell synapses beginning at 6–8 h following transient cerebral ischemia [17]. The timing and characteristics of the electrophysiological changes in the above studies closely resemble the L-PSPs observed in the present study. Moreover, a similar NMDA-receptor-mediated late synaptic response has been recorded in the CA1 region of hippocampal slices after blockade of $GABA_A$ receptors [28] or adenosine A1 receptors in normal conditions [29], or after an anoxic-aglycemic episode [22, 30], suggesting that an NMDA-receptor-mediated local excitatory network [31, 32] may be unmasked after ischemic insult.

In contrast to L-PSP neurons, non-L-PSP neurons failed to develop L-PSPs but displayed a depression of synaptic transmission following reperfusion. This ischemia-induced synaptic depression resembles the long-term depression (LTD) that has recently been described and widely studied in the CA1 region of hippocampus in vitro [33–35] and in vivo [36]. Depression of the synaptic transmission was also observed in S-EPSP neurons, but was quite different from that in non-L-PSP neurons. S-EPSP neurons appeared approximately 31 h after reperfusion with great depression of synaptic transmission when the depression of non-L-PSP neurons started to recover at this time point. In addition, the excitability of S-EPSP neurons progressively deteriorated, while the decrease of excitability in non-L-PSP neurons was transient. Therefore, depression of the synaptic transmission in S-EPSP neurons may be a sign of cell degeneration.

The gradual increase of the spike threshold in L-PSP and S-EPSP neurons indicates that neuronal excitability in these cells is progressively depressed following reperfusion. In contrast, only a transient increase in spike threshold was observed in non-L-PSP neurons. Using the gerbil brain slice preparation at different time points after ischemia, Urban et al. [18] reported that the excitability of CA1 neurons was depressed in a similar time-dependent fashion. The depression of neuronal excitability may be responsible for the decrease in spontaneous firing rate of CA1 neurons following ischemia, as observed in the present study and in previous reports [9–11, 37]. It has been shown that decreased excitability of CA1 neurons during anoxia is due to the increase in potassium conductance [13, 14, 38]. The mechanisms causing the increase of spike threshold in CA1 neurons after reperfusion are not yet clear.

Electrophysiological Changes and Selective Neuronal Damage following Ischemia

The present study has demonstrated that most of the CA1 neurons die 1 week after approximately 13 min of ID. After ischemia of the same severity, the number of L-PSP neurons progressively increased. The S-EPSP neurons appeared at the late time points following reperfusion. The excitability of L-PSP and S-EPSP neurons progressively deteriorated, whereas the excitability of non-L-PSP neurons transiently decreased, resembling what has been observed in CA1 neurons after sublethal ischemia [37]. Based on the above observations, it is conceivable that L-PSP and S-EPSP neurons are the degenerating neurons and non-L-PSP neurons are the surviving neurons after ischemic insult. Neurons with L-PSP may represent the early phase of post-ischemic cell damage, while neurons with S-EPSP may be in the late phase of cell degeneration. Another possibility is that L-PSP and non-L-PSP neurons may represent different types of cell degeneration following ischemia. It has been suggested that two different pathways exist in postischemic cell death: neurons with higher intracellular Ca^{2+} die fast and may be associated with necrotic cell death, while neurons with lower intracellular Ca^{2+} may undergo apoptotic cell death [39]. It is possible that L-PSP neurons undergo necrosis, and non-L-PSP neurons undergo apoptotic cell death following ischemia.

The ischemia-vulnerable and ischemia-resistant neurons displayed a completely different response to severe ischemia in terms of synaptic transmission: potentiation in CA1 neurons, and suppression in CA3 and granule cells. Because most of the CA1 neurons die after such severe ischemia, it is conceivable that enhancement of the synaptic transmission plays a role in postischemic cell death. On the other hand, depression of the synaptic transmission may be associated with mechanisms of survival after ischemia based on the following observations: (1) The synaptic transmission was transiently suppressed in CA3 neurons that survive severe ischemia, as shown in the present study, and (2) the synaptic transmission was also transiently suppressed in CA1 and CA3 neurons after mild sublethal ischemia [24, 37, 40]. If glutamate excitotoxicity plays a role in the pathogenesis of postischemic cell death, it probably acts on the enhancement of synaptic transmission, rather than increasing the neuronal firing rate. Further study is needed to elucidate how enhancement of the synaptic transmission following ischemia induces neuronal damage.

Acknowledgement

This research is supported by grants NS33103 and NS38053 from the NIH.

References

1 Graham DI: Hypoxia and vascular disorders; in Adams JH, Duchen LW (eds): Greenfild's Neuropathology, ed 5. London, Arnold, 1992, pp 161–198.
2 Pulsinelli WA: Selective neuronal vulnerability: Morphological and molecular characteristics. Prog Brain Res 1985;63:29–37.
3 Kirino T: Delayed neuronal death in gerbil hippocampus following ischemia. Brain Res 1982;237:57–69.
4 Pulsinelli WA, Brierley JB, Plum F: Temporal profile of neuronal damage in a model of transient forebrain ischemia. Ann Neurol 1982;11:491–498.
5 Choi DW, Rothman SM: The role of glutamate neurotoxicity in hypoxic-ischemic neuronal death. Annu Rev Neurosci 1990;13:171–182.
6 Rothman SM, Olney JW: Glutamate and the pathophysiology of hypoxic-ischemic brain damage. Ann Neurol 1986;19:105–111.
7 Chang HS, Sasaki T, Kassel NF: Hippocampal unit activity after transient ischemia in rats. Stroke 1989;20:1051–1058.
8 Suzuki R, Yamaguchi T, Li CL, Klatzo I: The effects of 5-minute ischemia in mongolian gerbils. II. Changes of spontaneous neuronal activity in cerebral cortex and CA1 sector of hippocampus. Acta Neuropathol (Berl) 1983;60:217–222.
9 Buzsáki G, Freund TF, Bayardo F, Somogyi P: Ischemia-induced changes in the electrical activity of the hippocampus. Exp Brain Res 1989;78:268–278.
10 Furukawa K, Yamana K, Kogure K: Postischemic alterations of spontaneous activities in rat hippocampal CA1 neurons. Brain Res 1990;530: 257–260.
11 Imon H, Mitani A, Andou Y, Arai T, Kataoka K: Delayed neuronal death is induced without postischemic hyperexcitability: Continuous multiple-unit recording from ischemic CA1 neurons. J Cereb Blood Flow Metab 1991;11:819–823.
12 Balestrino M, Aitken PG, Somjen GG: Spreading depression-like hypoxic depolarization in CA1 and fascia dentata of hippocampal slices: Relationship to selective vulnerability. Brain Res 1989;497:102–107.
13 Fujiwara N, Higashi H, Shimoji K, Yoshimura M: Effects of hypoxia on rat hippocampal neurons in vitro. J Physiol (Lond) 1987;384:131–151.
14 Hansen AJ, Hounsgaard J, Jahnsen H: Anoxia increases potassium conductance in hippocampal nerve cells. Acta Physiol Scand 1982;115: 301–310.
15 Hori N, Doi N, Miyahara S, Shinoda Y, Carpenter DO: Appearance of NMDA receptors triggered by anoxia independent of voltage in vivo and in vitro. Exp Neurol 1991;112: 304–311.
16 Kirino T, Robinson HPC, Miwa A, Tamura A, Kawai N: Disturbance of membrane function preceding ischemic delayed neuronal death in the gerbil hippocampus. J Cereb Blood Flow Metab 1992;12:408–417.

17 Miyazaki S, Katayama Y, Furuichi M, Kinoshita K, Kawamata T, Tsubokawa T: Post-ischemic potentiation of Schaffer collateral/CA1 pyramidal cell responses of the rat hippocampus in vivo: Involvement of N-methyl-*D*-aspartate receptors. Brain Res 1993;611:155–159.
18 Urban L, Neill K, Crain B, Nadler JV, Somjen G: Postischemic synaptic physiology in area CA1 of the gerbil hippocampus studied in vitro. J Neurosci 1989;9:3966–3975.
19 Jensen MS, Lambert JDC, Johansen FF: Elecrophysiological recordings from rat hippocampus slices following in vivo brain ischemia. Brain Res 1991;554:166–175.
20 Pulsinelli WA, Brierley JB: A new model of bilateral hemispheric ischemia in the unanesthetized rat. Stroke 1979;10:267–272.
21 Crépel V, Hammond C, Chinestra P, Diabira D, Ben-Ari YA: Selective LTP of NMDA receptor-mediated currents induced by anoxia in CA1 hippocampal neurons. J Neurophysiol 1993;70:2045–2055.
22 Crépel V, Ben-Ari Y: Intracellular injection of a Ca^{2+} chelator prevents generation of anoxic LTP. J Neurophysiol 1996;75:770–778.
23 Czéh G, Aitken PG, Somjen GG: Membrane currents in CA1 pyramidal cells during spreading depression (SD) and SD-like hypoxic depolarization. Brain Res 1993;632:195–208.
24 Xu ZC, Pulsinelli WA: Responses of CA1 pyramidal neurons in rat hippocampus to transient forebrain ischemia: An in vivo intracellular recording study. Neurosci Lett 1994; 171:187–191.
25 Hu BR, Wieloch T: Persistent translocation of Ca^{2+}/calmodulin-dependent protein kinase II to synaptic junctions in the vulnerable hippocampal CA1 region following transient ischemia. J Neurochem 1995; 64:277–284.
26 Roche KW, Tingley WG, Huganir RL: Glutamate receptor phosphorylation and synaptic plasticity. Curr Opin Neurobiol 1994;4:383–388.
27 Schulman H: Protein phosphorylation in neuronal plasticity and gene expression. Curr Opin Neurobiol 1995;5:375–381.
28 Crépel V, Khazipov R, Ben-Ari Y: Blocking $GABA_A$ inhibition reveals AMPA- and NMDA-receptor-mediated polysynaptic responses in the CA1 region of the rat hippocampus. J Neurophysiol 1997;77:2071–2082.
29 Klishin A, Tsintsadze T, Lozovaya N, Krishtal O: Latent N-methyl-*D*-aspartate receptors in the recurrent excitatory pathway between hippocampal CA1 pyramidal neurons: Ca^{2+}-dependent activation by blocking A1 adenosine receptors. Proc Natl Acad Sci USA 1995;92:12431–12435.
30 Tsintsadze T, Lozovaya N, Klishin A, Krishtal O: NMDA receptor-mediated synapses between CA1 neurons: Activation by ischaemia. Neuroreport 1996;7:2679–2682.
31 Deuchars J, Thomson AL: CA1 pyramid-pyramid connections in rat hippocampus in vitro: Dual intracellular recordings with biocytin filling. Neuroscience 1996;74:1009–1018.
32 Thomson AM, Radpou S: Excitatory connections between CA1 pyramidal cells revealed by spike triggered averaging in slices of rat hippocampus are partially NMDA receptor mediated. Eur J Neurosci 1991;3: 587–601.
33 Bear MF, Malenka RC: Synaptic plasticity: LTP and LTD. Curr Opin Neurobiol 1994;4:389–399.
34 Dudek SM, Bear MF: Homosynaptic long-term depression in area CA1 of the rat hippocampus and effects of N-methyl-*D*-aspartate receptor blockade. Proc Natl Acad Sci USA 1992;89:4363–4367.
35 Mulkey RM, Malenka RC: Mechanisms underlying induction of homosynaptic long-term depression in area CA1 of hippocampus. Neuron 1992;9:967–975.
36 Heynen AJ, Abraham WC, Bear MF: Bidirectional modification of CA1 synapse in the adult hippocampus in vivo. Nature 1996;381:163–166.
37 Xu ZC, Pulsinelli WA: Neurophysiological changes of CA1 pyramidal neurons following transient ischemia: An in vivo intracellular recording and staining study. J Neurophysiol 1996;76:1689–1697.
38 Lebond J, Krenjevic K: Hypoxic changes in hippocampal neurons. J Neurophysiol 1989;62:1–14.
39 Choi DW: Ischemia-induced neuronal apoptosis. Curr Opin Neurobiol 1996;6:667–672.
40 Howard EM, Gao TM, Pulsinelli WA, Xu ZC: Electrophysiological changes of CA3 neurons and dentate granule cells following transient forebrain ischemia. Brain Res 1998; 798:109–118.

Biological Signals and Receptors

Biol Signals Recept 1999;8:309–315

Received: November 20, 1998
Accepted: December 4, 1998

Involvement of K^+ Channels in the Inhibitory Effects of Adenosine on Anoxia-Induced $[Ca^{2+}]_i$ Increase in Cultured Rat Hippocampal CA1 Neurons

Qin Wan Hang Yao Fu-Zhuang Wang

Department of Neurobiology, Institute of Basic Medical Sciences, Academy of Military Medical Sciences, Beijing, China

Key Words
Adenosine · Anoxia · $[Ca^{2+}]_i$ · Potassium channels · Confocal laser scanning microscope · Hippocampal neurons

Abstract
Changes in intracellular free Ca^{2+} concentration ($[Ca^{2+}]_i$) in cultured hippocampal CA1 neurons isolated from newborn rats were measured by a confocal laser scanning microscope, using the Ca^{2+} indicator Fluo-3. The results showed that exogenous adenosine (100 μ*M*) significantly attenuated the increase of neuronal $[Ca^{2+}]_i$ induced by acute anoxia. This effect of adenosine could be suppressed by the adenosine A1 receptor antagonist 8-cyclopentyltheophylline. Moreover, potassium channel blockers, aminopyridine, and glipizide could also block the inhibitory role of adenosine, but tetraethylammonium had no effect. These results suggest that adenosine may activate 4-AP or ATP-sensitive potassium channels via an A1-receptor-mediated mechanism and consequently inhibit anoxia-induced $[Ca^{2+}]_i$ elevation in hippocampal neurons.

Introduction

Cerebral anoxia is an important pathological condition which leads to an irreversible cerebral dysfunction and extensive death of neurons. It has been believed that anoxia can induce an overload of cytosolic Ca^{2+}, which is regarded as the major cause resulting in neuronal damage and death [1, 2].

Adenosine (ADO) is now widely accepted as the major inhibitory neuromodulator in the central nervous system, which can provide a

KARGER
Fax + 41 61 306 12 34
E-Mail karger@karger.ch
www.karger.com

1422–4933/99/0085–0309$17.50/0

Accessible online at:
http://BioMedNet.com/karger

Fu-Zhuang Wang
Institute of Basic Medical Sciences
P.O. Box 130(3)
Beijing 100850 (China)

homeostatic regulation between the energy metabolic state of neurons and their excitability [3]. Previous researchers have demonstrated that ADO is normally present in extracellular fluid at concentrations of about 1 μM and is released in increased amounts during periods of anoxia, ischemia or intense neuronal activity [4, 5]. In the hippocampus, ADO has been known to produce several effects, including a presynaptic decrease of neurotransmitter release, enhancement of K^+ conductance and membrane hyperpolarization [6, 7]. In addition, ADO can also inhibit postsynaptic neuronal Ca^{2+} influx [8]. However, the exact mechanism underlying this inhibitory role of ADO, and especially the question whether K^+ channels are involved in the actions of ADO, still remain unknown. In the present study, the confocal laser scanning microscope, in conjunction with the Ca^{2+}-sensitive fluorescent probe Fluo-3, was used to record the changes in intracellular free calcium concentrations ($[Ca^{2+}]_i$) in cultured hippocampal CA1 neurons in response to anoxia. Based on this model, the effect of ADO, and particularly the role of several K^+ channels in the mechanism of ADO, were examined.

Materials and Methods

Cell Cultures

The hippocampus was isolated from newborn Wistar rats, and the CA1 layer was separated under a dissecting microscope. The tissue was incubated at 37 °C in 0.125% trypsin for 30 min, and then dissociated by gentle passage through the tip of a frame-narrowed Pasteur pipette, and plated in 35-mm collagen-coated tissue culture plates (Falon) at a density of 5×10^5 cells/ml. The plates were kept in a 37 °C incubator in humidified atmosphere containing 10% CO_2 in air. The medium contained 94% Eagle's MEM, 5% horse serum, 1% nutrient supplement and 100 µg/ml glutamine [9]. On day 5, cytarabine (3 µg/ml) was added to inhibit further growth of nonneuronal cells. Cultures were fed twice a week by replacing 50% of the medium with fresh medium.

Loading Cells with Fluo-3

Experiments were performed on 14-day-cultured CA1 pyramidal-like neurons. Prior to measurements, cells were bathed in recording medium with Fluo-3/AM (5 μM) dye in the presence of Pluronic F-127 (0.075%), and incubated at room temperature sheltered from light for 30–60 min. Before use, cells were washed with normal recording medium.

Recording of Intracellular Calcium

An Ultima/ACAS 212 confocal laser scanning microscope (Meridian Instrument, USA) was used to measure the transient change of neuronal $[Ca^{2+}]_i$. Fluo-3 emission was induced by the 488 nm band of the Ar-Kr laser and detected by a photomultiplier tube at a wavelength of 515 nm. The Ca^{2+} fluorescent images around some areas were recorded, and a line was drawn to reveal the changes in fluorescence responses to anoxia or drug application. Anoxia was induced by perfusing 95% N_2 + 5% CO_2 into the recording medium, and drugs were applied by pressure ejection. Data were presented as the percentage of the peak amplitude (F_{max}) induced by anoxia or drug application to the baseline (F_0) in fluorescent intensity of neuronal $[Ca^{2+}]_i$ (mean ± SEM), and $\Delta f(\%) = (F_{max} - F_0)/F_0 \times 100\%$ was determined, where Δf is normalized change with respect to the baseline.

Solutions and Drugs

The recording medium contained (in mM): 150 NaCl, 5 KCl, 7 $CaCl_2$, 1 $MgCl_2$, 6 glucose and 10 HEPES, and pH was adjusted to 7.3. ADO, the ADO A1 receptor agonist N^6-cyclohexyladenosine (CHA), the antagonist 8-cyclopentyltheophylline (CPT), the potassium channel blockers tetraethylammonium (TEA) and aminopyridine (4-AP), as well as the ATP-sensitive potassium channel blocker glipizide (GLI) were all obtained from Sigma Chemical Comapny. Fluo-3/AM and Pluronic F-127 were from Sigma, too. They were prepared in dimethylsulfoxide and stored at –20 °C.

Results

Response of Hippocampal CA1 Neurons to Anoxia

Cultured rat hippocampal CA1 neurons were found to respond rapidly to anoxia. Within 50–60 s (56 ± 16, n = 6) of anoxic exposure, these neurons showed a sharp in-

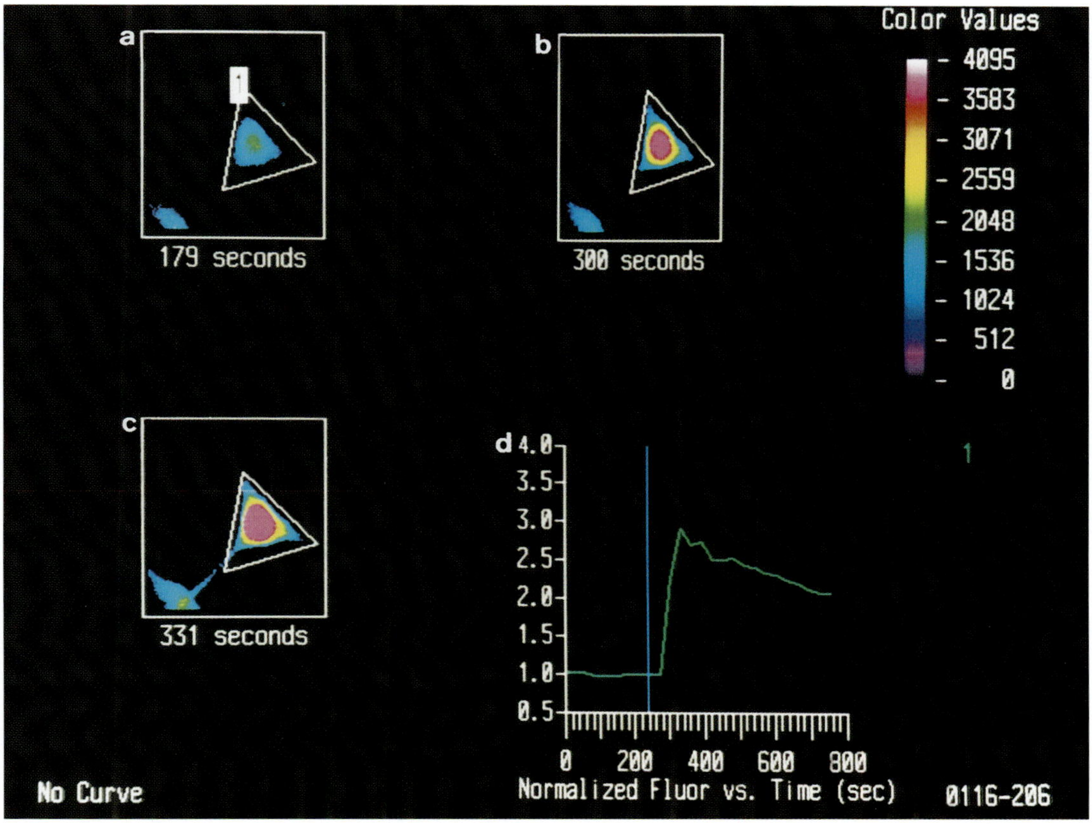

Fig. 1. The anoxia-induced increase of $[Ca^{2+}]_i$ in cultured rat hippocampal CA1 neurons. Images of the Fluo-3 fluorescence from a 14-day-cultured CA1 neuron before and after anoxia were taken by a confocal microscope. The scale ranging from violet (low $[Ca^{2+}]_i$) to white (high $[Ca^{2+}]_i$) is shown in the vertical spectrum. **a** Taken during baseline recording before anoxia; **b**, **c** taken several minutes after exposure to anoxia; **d** $[Ca^{2+}]$ curve of normalized fluor vs time. Blue bar indicates the start of anoxia.

crease in intracellular free Ca^{2+}, as demonstrated by increased Fluo-3 fluorescence (fig. 1). The maximum percentage increase in fluorescence was 235 ± 88% (n = 6).

Effect of ADO on Anoxia-Induced Increase of $[Ca^{2+}]_i$ in Hippocampal Neurons

In hippocampal neurons, the baseline fluorescence remained unchanged when 100 μ*M* of ADO was applied exogenously. These neurons exhibited a much slower and smaller increase in fluorescence in response to anoxia than normal controls, as shown in the example of figure 2. The percentage increase in contrast to baseline $[Ca^{2+}]_i$ after exposure to anoxia for 10 min is only 53 ± 31% (n = 10), which is significantly lower than the response of CA1 neurons to anoxia in the absence of ADO ($p < 0.05$). Moreover, the latency of the onset of rise in fluorescence (measured from baseline to peak) was also significantly longer than that of the controls. When the ADO A1

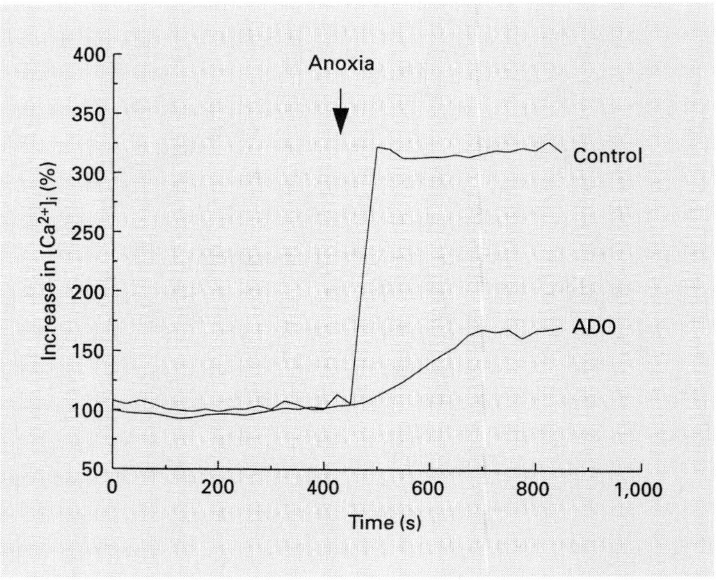

Fig. 2. ADO inhibition of anoxia-induced $[Ca^{2+}]_i$ elevation in cultured hippocampal CA1 neurons. The two curves recorded from two different cells show the changes of $[Ca^{2+}]_i$ for one in normal solution and one in the presence of 100 µ*M* of ADO.

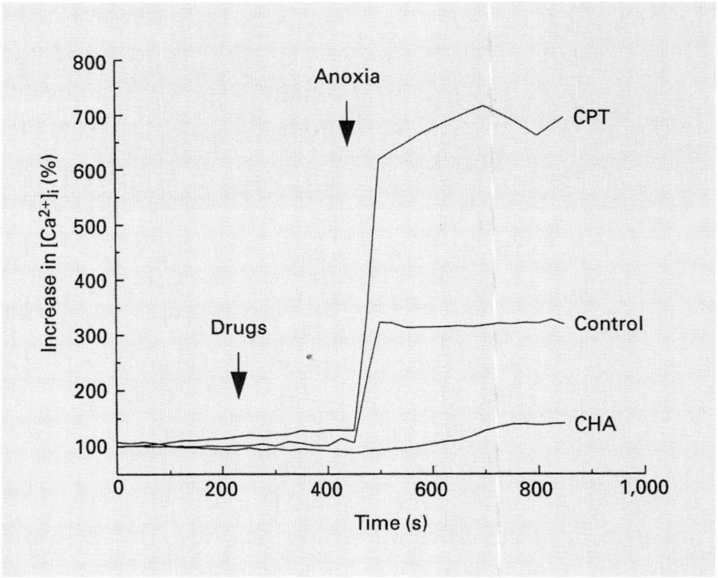

Fig. 3. Effects of the ADO A1 receptor agonist or antagonist on $[Ca^{2+}]_i$ in cultured hippocampal CA1 neurons during anoxia. Three curves recorded from three different cells show the changes of $[Ca^{2+}]_i$ for one in normal solution and the other two in the presence of CHA (20 µ*M*) and CPT (20 µ*M*), respectively.

receptor agonist CHA (20 µ*M*) was added in advance, anoxia only elicited a fluorescence increase of approximately 44% (n = 5), similar to that of ADO. But when neurons were exposed to 20 µ*M* of CPT, the selective antagonist of the ADO A1 receptor, they had a markedly different response to the same anoxic condition. In a sample of five cells, the rise in neuronal $[Ca^{2+}]_i$ was 502 ± 189% (n = 5), which is significantly higher than in normal anoxic controls (fig. 3). These results demonstrate that exogenous ADO can signifi-

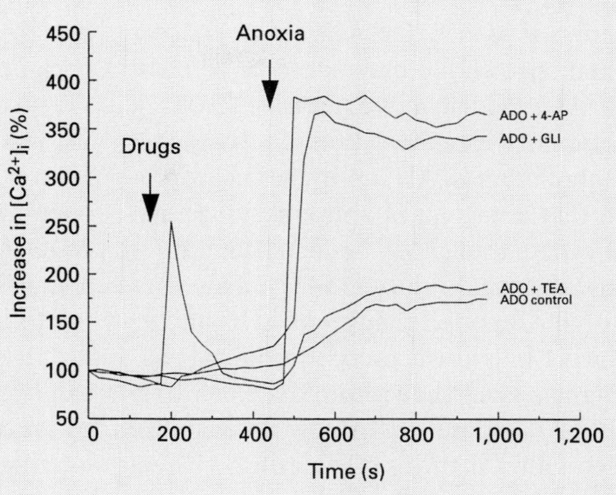

Fig. 4. Effects of K^+ channel blockers on the inhibitory role of ADO in anoxia-induced $[Ca^{2+}]_i$ elevation in cultured hippocampal CA1 neurons. Four curves recorded from four different cells show the changes of $[Ca^{2+}]_i$ for one in normal solution and the other three in the presence of TEA (10 m*M*) + ADO (100 μ*M*), 4-AP (1 m*M*) + ADO (100 μ*M*), and GLI (20 μ*M*) + ADO (100 μ*M*), respectively.

cantly inhibit $[Ca^{2+}]_i$ increase induced by anoxia in hippocampal CA1 neurons through the activation of A1 receptors.

Effects of Several K^+ Channel Blockers on the Inhibitory Role of ADO in Anoxia-Induced $[Ca^{2+}]_i$ Increase

In order to determine whether the inhibitory role of ADO on anoxia-induced $[Ca^{2+}]_i$ increase is related to the activation of K^+ channels, three different types of K^+ channel blockers, TEA, 4-AP and GLI, were applied prior to the addition of 100 μ*M* of ADO, and anoxia was performed subsequently. The application of TEA (10 m*M*) caused a transient rise in neuronal $[Ca^{2+}]_i$, and then a rapid recovery to the baseline level. During anoxia, these neurons only exhibited a slight rise in $[Ca^{2+}]_i$ (75 ± 22%, n = 5), similar to the response when only ADO was applied. When 4-AP (1 m*M*) and GLI (20 μ*M*) were added, respectively, no changes in fluorescence were observed. But after anoxia, neuronal $[Ca^{2+}]_i$ produced drastic increases of 266 ± 91% (n = 5) and 437 ± 229% (n = 5), respectively, markedly different from the changes in the presence of ADO only (fig. 4).

Discussion

Among the theories of neuronal damage induced by anoxia, one of the most widely considered is excitatory amino acid (EAA) neurotoxicity and intracellular Ca^{2+} overload. Anoxia induces a drastic release of presynaptic EAA, which results in an excessive membrane depolarization of neurons. This initiates several vicious circles which may lead to an uncontrolled neuronal Ca^{2+} loading [10, 11]. For example, depolarization favors Ca^{2+} influx through voltage-dependent Ca^{2+} channels, and by removing the voltage-sensitive Mg^{2+} blockade, it also allows Ca^{2+} to enter through NMDA-receptor-operated Ca^{2+} channels [12, 13]. The resulting neuronal overload of Ca^{2+} is thought to play a key role in the initiation and further escalation of the pathological process which finally leads to anoxic nerve cell death [14].

There is evidence that ADO is an endogenous neuroprotective metabolite in cerebral anoxia. As a mediator of a negative feedback interaction between the neuronal activity and its metabolic states, ADO provides neuroprotection that antagonizes a number of pathological events thought to be instrumental for ischemic neuronal injury [15–17]. This is in line with the reported changes of ADO and its receptor A1 in hypoxic preconditioning [18].

ADO has been shown to reduce neuronal Ca^{2+} influx [19], but up to now no evidence has been found that this effect exerts a direct action on Ca^{2+} channels in hippocampal pyramidal neurons. Neither transient nor long-lasting types of Ca^{2+} currents appear to be affected by ADO [20, 21]. For this reason, we suppose that the reduction in Ca^{2+} influx by ADO observed in our experiments results from the increase of ADO-mediated K^+ conductance. So several different types of K^+ channel blockers were applied to test and verify this hypothesis.

Our results indicate that the potassium channel blockers 4-AP and GLI could abolish the inhibitory role of ADO in the anoxia-induced increase of neuronal $[Ca^{2+}]_i$, suggesting a close relationship between the effect of ADO on $[Ca^{2+}]_i$ change during anoxia and the activation of K^+ channels. 4-AP- or ATP-sensitive K^+ channels seem to be involved in the mechanism of action of ADO on neuronal Ca^{2+} influx induced by anoxia.

On the other hand, since the ADO A1 receptor antagonist CPT can seriously aggravate the neuronal $[Ca^{2+}]_i$-increasing tendency, we conclude that endogenous ADO is markedly released in hippocampal neurons during anoxia. Through acting on its A1 receptors, it results in the decreased cytosolic Ca^{2+} level and consequently plays a protective role against neuronal injury.

All these results show that the inhibitory role of ADO in the increase of neuronal $[Ca^{2+}]_i$ induced by anoxia in cultured rat hippocampal CA1 neurons is related to the activation of 4-AP- or ATP-sensitive K^+ channels via an A1-receptor-mediated mechanism. How does ADO decrease $[Ca^{2+}]_i$ through the opening of K^+ channels? We assume that ADO may activate 4-AP- or ATP-sensitive K^+ channels through coupling A1 receptors, leading to intracellular K^+ outflow and hyperpolarization of the neuronal membrane, which can resist the excessive depolarization evoked by anoxia. As a consequence of this hyperpolarizing effect, neuronal Ca^{2+} influx is greatly decreased through voltage-dependent Ca^{2+} channels as well as through NMDA-receptor-operated Ca^{2+} channels by the maintenance of a voltage-sensitive Mg^{2+} block. In this way, ADO can antagonize a cascade of cytotoxic events mediated by excessive intracellular Ca^{2+}, thus resulting in neuronal damage, and consequently play an important neuroprotective role against anoxia.

Acknowledgment

This project was supported by the National Natural Science Foundation of China (No. 39470601).

References

1 Lipton P, Lobner D: Mechanisms of intracellular calcium accumulation in the CA1 region of rat hippocampus during anoxia in vitro. Stroke 1990;21(suppl III):60–64.
2 Choi DW: Calcium-mediated neurotoxicity: Relationship to specific channel types and role in ischemic damage. Trends Neurosci 1988;11:465–469.
3 Deckert J, Gleiter CH: Adenosine – an endogenous neuroprotective metabolite and neuromodulator. J Neural Transm 1994;43(suppl):23–31.
4 Pedata F, Latini S, Pugliese AM, Pepeu G: Investigations into the adenosine outflow from hippocampal slices evoked by ischemia-like conditions. J Neurochem 1993;16:284–289.
5 Johansson AW, Fredholm BB: Release of adenosine and other purines from hippocampal slices stimulated electrically or by hypoxia/hypoglycemia. Life Science 1994;55:721–728.
6 Heron A, Lasbennes F, Seylaz J: Adenosine modulation of amino acid release in rat hippocampus during ischemia and veratridine depolarization. Brain Res 1993;608:27–32.
7 Dunwiddie TV, Fredholm BB: Adenosine A1 receptors inhibit adenylate cyclase activity and neurotransmitter release and hyperpolarize pyramidal neurons in rat hippocampus. J Pharmacol Exp Ther 1989;249:31–37.
8 Thompson SM, Haas HL, Gahwiler BH: Comparison of the actions of adenosine at pre- and postsynaptic receptors in the rat hippocampus in vitro. J Physiol Lond 1992;451:347–363.
9 Ding AS, Wang FZ: The growth characteristics of newborn rat hippocampal neurons in serum-free media. Chin J Cell Biol 1993;15:88–90.
10 Choi DW, Hartley DM: Calcium- and glutamate-induced cortical neuronal death; in Waxman SG (ed): Molecular and Cellular Approaches to the Treatment of Neurological Disease. New York, Raven Press, pp 23–24.
11 Frandsen A, Schousboe A: Excitatory amino-acid-mediated cytotoxicity and calcium homeostasis in cultured neurons. J Neurochem 1993;60:1202–1211.
12 Rudolphi KA, Schubert P, Parkinson FE, Fredholm BB: Neuroprotective role of adenosine in cerebral ischemia. Trends Pharmacol Sci 1992;13:439–445.
13 Schubert P, Rudolphi KA, Fredholm BB, Nakamura Y: Modulation of nerve and glial function by adenosine – role in the development of ischemic damage. Int J Biochem 1994;26:1227–1236.
14 Nicotera P, Orrenius S: Ca^{2+} and cell death. Ann NY Acad Sci 1992;648:17–27.
15 Phillis JW, O'Regan MH: Prevention of ischemic brain injury by adenosine receptor activation. Drug Dev Res 1993;28:390–394.
16 Lee KS, Lowenkopf T: Endogenous adenosine delays the onset of hypoxic depolarization in the rat hippocampus in vitro via an action at A1 receptors. Brain Res 1993;609:313–315.
17 Abbracchio MP, Brambilla R, Camisa M, et al: Adenosine A1 receptors in rat brain synaptosomes: Transductional mechanisms, effects on glutamate release and preservation after metabolic inhibition. Drug Dev Res 1995;35:119–129.
18 Zhang WL, Lu GW: Changes of adenosine and its A_1 receptor in hypoxic preconditioning. Biol Signals Recept 1999;8:275–280.
19 Andine P: Involvement of adenosine in ischemic and postischemic calcium regulation. Mol Chem Neuropathol 1993;18:35–49.
20 Salter MW, Koninck YD, Henry JL: Physiological roles for adenosine and ATP in synaptic transmission in the spinal dorsal horn. Prog Neurobiol 1993;41:125–156.
21 Haas HL, Gerber U, Greene RW, Stevens DR: Electrophysiological analysis of exogenous and endogenous adenosine actions in the rat and human hippocampus in vitro. Drug Dev Res 1993;28:386–389.

Biological Signals and Receptors

Biol Signals Recept 1999;8:316–322

Received: November 13, 1998
Accepted: December 1, 1998

Protective Effects of Intermittent Hypoxic Adaptation on Myocardium and Its Mechanisms

Jian-Guo Zhuang Zhao-Nian Zhou

Shanghai Institute of Physiology, Chinese Academy of Sciences, Shanghai, China

Key Words
Cardioprotection · Intermittent hypoxia · Adaptation · Myocardium

Abstract
Intermittent hypoxic adaptation offers as many beneficial effects in protecting against myocardial injuries as chronic continuous hypoxic adaptation. However, chronic continuous hypoxic adaptation readily causes some adverse effects on the organism, which may be prevented by intermittent hypoxic adaptation. As an approach to potentiate the protective effects, intermittent hypoxic adaptation is also much easier to apply to subjects who are not living at high altitude. The mechanisms underlying the cardioprotective effects of intermittent hypoxic adaptation are less understood, although great similarities exist between chronic continuous and intermittent hypoxic adaptation. The participation of several factors, such as myocardial vascularity, coronary blood flow, and cardiomyoglobin, which comprise the oxygen uptake system is not apparent, while the more efficient energetic metabolism after intermittent hypoxic adaptation may be a mechanism for cardioprotection. The possible roles of several signaling transduction pathways, including adrenoceptors, prostaglandins, and the adenosinergic system, in the beneficial effects of intermittent hypoxia are compared to those of chronic continuous hypoxic adaptation. Antioxidant enzymes and stress proteins may also be part of the mechanisms contributing to the cardioprotection of the intermittent hypoxic adaptation. As the cardioprotective effects of intermittent hypoxic adaptation employ multifold mechanisms, their clear elucidation needs more efforts.

KARGER

Fax + 41 61 306 12 34
E-Mail karger@karger.ch
www.karger.com

1422–4933/99/0085–0316$17.50/0

Accessible online at:
http://BioMedNet.com/karger

Prof. Zhao-Nian Zhou
Shanghai Institute of Physiology, Chinese Academy of Sciences
320 Yue-Yang Road
Shanghai 200031 (China)
Tel. +86 21 64313251 8500, Fax +86 21 64746305

Introduction

It has been known for many years that the long-term adaptive process of high-altitude hypoxia can increase the resistance of the heart against injury. Most of those experimental investigations were carried out through clinical-epidemiological observations in the late fifties, and found that the incidence of myocardial infarction and mortality from coronary heart disease is significant reduced in high-altitude residents [1, 2]. However, chronic continuous high-altitude hypoxic acclimatization, especially in lowlanders, may also exert adverse effects, such as polycythemia, right ventricular hypertrophy, and heart failure [3]. On the contrary, intermittent hypoxic adaptation can also offer cardioprotection against injurious factors [4–6] and is beneficial to a variety of physical illnesses and mental disorders, such as ischemic heart disease [7], while adverse effects can be limited to the lowest degree [8]. Furthermore, it is much easier to apply intermittent instead of continuous hypoxia to humans not living at high altitude. Therefore, potential applications of intermittent hypoxic adaptation for clinical and prophylactic purposes are apparent. As a result, the exploration of the mechanism of intermittent hypoxic adaptation has drawn much attention in the last three decades [8], although the mechanism of cardioprotection is still far from clear. Differences in the mechanisms of action between adaptation to continuous and to intermittent hypoxia have been well described by Meerson [7] in 1993. The mechanisms of chronic continuous hypoxic adaptation have been well discussed by Kolar [9]. This review will focus on some proposed mechanisms concerning the cardioprotective effects of intermittent hypoxic adaptation in the myocardium per se discussed in the studies of recent years.

Oxygen Uptake

Myocardial microvessels, coronary flow and cardiac myoglobin are the substantial bases for oxygen transportation from blood to the mitochondria in the myocardium. They are therefore likely to play important parts in the protective effects on myocardium offered by intermittent hypoxic adaptation.

Myocardial Vascularity and Coronary Blood Flow

It is likely that chronic continuous hypoxia acts as a stimulus for the growth of additional microvessels in the myocardium. The mechanical effects due to chronic increases in coronary blood flow, as well as the hypoxia-induced formation and release of angiogenic growth factors, such as vascular endothelial growth factor, may play a role in coronary angiogenesis [10]. However, studies concerning the coronary capillary density in animals adapted to high altitude have not yielded an unequivocal result [11]. Much less studies have focused on the myocardial vascularity and coronary flow under intermittent hypoxic conditions. Limited observations [12] showed that the capillary density and related capillary domain area, the capillary tissue supply unit and the index of heterogeneity of capillary spacing were not significantly changed in the heart of rats undergoing intermittent hypoxic adaptation. Therefore, it seems that myocardial vascularity and coronary flow are not those parts in the mechanism of cardioprotection by intermittent or continuous hypoxic adaptation, although their contribution to the beneficial effects needs clarification.

Myoglobin

Myoglobin serves as an intracellular reservoir and an oxygen shuttle in the myocardium of mammals. Numerous studies have evidenced an increase of myoglobin concentration as a result of chronic continuous hypoxia [1, 13]. However, the alterations of cardiac myoglobin concentrations under intermittent hypoxia have not been well studied. Accelerated myoglobin expression of cultured neonatal rat cardiac myocytes was observed with prolonged hypoxic exposure (48 h), and restoration of the expression occurred after 24 h of reoxygenation [14]. One recent study [13] showed that intermittent hypoxia (6 h/day, a total of 42 exposures up to hypobaric 3,500 m) did not change the myoglobin concentration of either the left or right ventricular myocardium in the rat. The authors simply attributed the absence of a significant myoglobin elevation to the good hypoxic adaptation of the rats. It is possible, however, that the hypoxic severity did not reach the threshold to trigger a stably accelerated myoglobin expression. Furthermore, as in chronic continuous hypoxic adaptation, significant differences between species or ages may also influence the cardiac myoglobin level in the intermittent hypoxic adaptation process. Even so, this study did not imply that myoglobin was a proposed mechanism in the cardioprotection offered by intermittent hypoxic adaptation.

Energetic Metabolism

Chronic continuous hypoxic adaptation is associated with a variety of adaptive changes at the level of myocardial energy production and utilization that enable the heart to work more economically and thus can protect the myocardium from the lack of oxygen. According to Moret [1], these changes may involve an increased capacity of aerobic metabolism, as indicated by the larger number of mitochondria, as well as enhanced activities of certain mitochondrial enzymes or cytochromes, an improved ability of mitochondria-generated energy in the presence of low ADP concentrations, greater efficiency of oxidative phosphorylation, and preferential use of the carbohydrates as substrate. An increased glycolytic capacity is also implied in the protective effect of acclimatization to high-altitude continuous hypoxia [15]. Chronic hypoxia decreases the specific activities of several sarcolemmal ATPases in the myocardium, and also increases their affinity for ATP [16]. This may elevate the efficiency of available ATP utilization and therefore help preserve membrane transport functions under conditions of low energy production. There are only few experiments especially designed to examine the effects of intermittent hypoxic adaptation on the process of energy metabolism. Kopylov et al. [17] checked the effect of intermittent hypoxic adaptation (hypobaric 4,000 m, 4 h daily × 40 days) on the resistance of the myocardial energy metabolism and contractile function to acute anoxia and subsequent reoxygenation. They found that adaptation to hypoxia significantly accelerated the restoration of creatine phosphate, ATP and creatine phosphokinase activity in myocardium in reoxygenation following acute anoxia. The reduction in oxygen consumption in the hearts of humans and animals undergoing continuous or intermittent hypoxic adaptation, as compared to control hearts [7], also supports the more efficient energy metabolic system being involved in the cardioprotective effects of intermittent hypoxic adaptation.

Adrenoceptor Responsiveness

Adaptation to chronic continuous hypoxia is characterized by a reduced β-adrenoceptor responsiveness [18] due to the downregulation of myocardial β-adrenoceptors [19]. Catecholamine degradation may also be enhanced in this situation, as indicated by the elevated activity of catechol-*o*-methyltransferase [20]. Those changes might be antiarrhythmic and cardioprotective when considering that they decrease the oxygen demand of the myocardium and increase the myocardial tolerance to toxic doses of isoprenaline [21]. Intermittent hypoxic adaptation is in a similar way affecting the myocardial adrenoceptors, as suggested by Burtscher et al. [22]. They showed that 4 weeks of interval hypoxic training lowered the heart rates and ventilation at submaximal workloads, without, however, diminishing maximum heart rates and performance.

Antioxidant Enyzmes

It is known that oxygen-derived free radicals are an important factor contributing to the ischemia/reperfusion- and hypoxia/reoxygenation-induced sarcolemmal damage to the myocardium. Endogenous antioxidant systems, such as superoxide dismutase and catalase, prevent the activation of the lipid perioxidant chain reaction and thus enhance the resistance of the myocardium to ischemia- or hypoxia-induced injury. Reoxygenation, rather than hypoxia, facilitates the generation of oxygen-derived free radicals. Because the apparent difference between continuous and intermittent hypoxic adaptation is the adaptive course of the latter, not only as a hypoxic session by itself but also being separated by several reoxygenation sessions, it is attractive to speculate that the reoxygenation sessions of intermittent hypoxic adaptation boost antioxidant generation in the cardiac tissue, and therefore protect the myocardium from later injury caused by oxygen-derived free radicals. Experimental evidence provided by Meerson [7] indicates that continuous hypoxia decreases the activity of the principal antioxidant enzymes in the heart, while intermittent hypoxia increases the enzymes. A recent study by Chen et al. [13] also showed elevated levels of antioxidant enzymes in the myocardium of rats undergoing 6 weeks of intermittent hypoxic adaptation (hypobaric 3,500 m, 6 h/day). However, they were unable to reveal any significant change of antioxidant enzyme activity in the myocardium of rats undergoing 4 weeks of adaptation. Also, in another study [23], no appreciable change in myocardial total antioxidant concentration was found in a similar model of chronic hypoxia. The importance of increased antioxidants in the mechanism of cardioprotective effects, therefore, needs to be re-examined. However, the different responses of antioxidants to continuous and intermittent hypoxic adaptation are definite, according to Meerson's [24] description. Increased antioxidant activity induced by intermittent hypoxic adaptation seems to be more involved in the protection of other organs like brain and liver.

Stress Proteins

Stress proteins or heat shock proteins (hsp) seem to be related to the enhancement of the tolerance of the myocardium to subsequent injurious stress. Acute hypoxia, like many other stimuli, induces the synthesis of stress proteins in isolated myocytes [25] and in the heart in vivo [26]. But it is not clear whether stress proteins play a role in the myocardial protection offered by chronic hypoxic adaptation, although it is attractive to think that their protective effects may be more pronounced in this case. But limited studies provide little agreement with this presumption. Acclimatization of rats to intermittent hypoxic exposure (40 days at a high altitude of 4,000 m) increased two hsp70 isoforms, but the resistance of the isolated perfused heart to postischemic contractile dysfunction and creatine kinase release was not improved [27]. In another study [28], two weeks of exposure to a simulated altitude of 5,000 m did not affect the expression of hsp70 mRNA in the heart. Therefore, the effects of stress proteins on the myocardial protection induced by chronic continuous and intermittent hypoxia need to be further studied.

Prostaglandins

Prostaglandins are capable of restricting and modulating the activation of the adrenergic link of stress reaction, and thus protecting the heart and other organs from injurious factors. Their antiarrhythmic effect, especially that of prostacyclin, has been well documented by Parratt [29]. Acute hypoxia significantly increases the production of prostaglandins in the myocardium [30]. With prolonged stay at a high altitude of 4,350 m, however, the plasma levels of those substances in humans return to control values after 8 days [31]. Intermittent hypoxic adaptation to a similar altitude (hypobaric-chamber-simulated) elevated the levels of prostaglandins in the myocardium of rats, remaining high even after 40 days of acclimatization [32]. A recent study [33] examined the possibility whether prostacyclin contributes to the cardioprotection provided by intermittent hypoxic adaptation. It was found that a single dose of 7-oxo-prostacyclin similarly increased the tolerance of isolated heart muscle to postanoxic contractile dysfunction in control and adapted rats. The protective effects of adaptation and prostacyclin were additive, suggesting that mechanisms other than prostaglandin involvement contribute to the cardioprotection offered by intermittent hypoxic adaptation.

Adenosinergic System

The formation of adenosine has been associated with a deficit of creatine phosphate and ATP, enhanced oxygen consumption in the cells, such as physical load and action of catecholamines, and insufficient oxygen supply, as under conditions of ischemia and hypoxia [24]. The protective effects of adenosine may involve many possible mechanisms, which have been reviewed in detail in a special issue of *Cardiovascular Research* [34]. Its release from the heart during acute hypoxia is also well documented. However, there is little information available about the possible involvement of the adenosinergic system in the cardioprotective effects of chronic hypoxic acclimatization. A recent study [35] shows that the prolonged exposure of rats to simulated high altitude decreases myocardial A_1 adenosine receptor density without any change in affinity for the agonist. Because adenosine is known to antagonize many effects of catecholamine, the reduced A_1 adenosine receptor density may thereby protect the heart against excessive stimulation of β-adrenoceptors. No direct evidence, however, is available at present to demonstrate that the adenosinergic system really takes part in any of the cardioprotective effects of chronic hypoxic acclimatization, either continuous or intermittent.

Other Possible Mechanisms

Apart from the mechanisms discussed above, there are several additional factors that may play possible roles in the beneficial effects offered by intermittent hypoxic adaptation. Bradykinin and nitric oxide, for example, have been suggested to act as endogenous myocardial protective mediators under certain circumstances [36], although their possible roles in mediating the cardioprotective effects of chronic continuous and intermittent hypoxic adaptation have not yet been examined. The enlargement in the size of cardiac myocytes is frequently reported in the chronically hypoxia-adapted species, including humans. But this is not the case in rats chronically adapted to inermittent hypoxia [12].

Conclusion

There seems to be sufficient evidence that intermittent hypoxic adaptation has a variety of protective effects, including cardioprotection, which have been well documented by Meerson [7, 24]. Also, its importance for clinical and prophylactic application is apparent, especially in the preconditioning of ischemic heart diseases. Even though there have been a great number of study results demonstrating neurohumoral alterations exerting fundamental influences on the cardioprotective effects offered by intermittent hypoxic adaptation [7, 24], the mechanisms underlying the cardioprotective effects mediated by the myocardium per se are still unclear. Limited studies suggest great similarities between chronic continuous and intermittent hypoxic adaptation in the different proposed mechanisms of cardioprotection, though there exist discrepancies between the two different patterns of hypoxic adaptation. Much more attention should be paid to ensuring the elucidation of possible mechanisms in the future.

References

1 Moret PR: Hypoxia and the heart; in Bourne GH (ed): Hearts and Heart-Like Organs. New York, Academic Press, 1980, pp 333–387.

2 Heath D, Williams DR: Man at High Altitude. Edinburgh, Churchill Livingstone, 1981.

3 Pei SX, Chen XJ, Si Ren BZ, Liu YH, Cheng XS, Harris EM, Harris PC: Chronic mountain sickness in Tibet. Q J Med 1989;266:555–574.

4 McGrath JJ, Prochazka J, Pelouch V, Ostadal B: Physiological responses of rats to intermittent high altitude stress. Effect of age. J Appl Physiol 1973;34:289–293.

5 Widimsky J, Urbanova D, Ressl J, Ostadal B, Pelouch V, Prochazka J: Effect of intermittent altitude hypoxia on the myocardium and lesser circulation in the rat. Cardiovasc Res 1973;7:798–808.

6 Meerson FZ, Ustinova EE, Manukhina EB: Prevention of cardiac arrhythmias by adaptation to hypoxia: Regulatory mechanisms and cardiotropic effect. Biomed Bichim Acta 1989;48(2–3):s83–88.

7 Meerson FZ: Essentials of Adaptive Medicine: Protective Effects of Adaptation (a Manual). Moscow, Hypoxia Medical, 1993.

8 Chen M, Zou ZN: The study on the protection of intermittent hypoxia in myocardium. Chin Bull Life Sci 1996;8:38–40.

9 Kolar F: Cardioprotective effects of hypoxia: Relation to preconditioning; in Wainwright CL, Parratt JR (eds): Myocardial Preconditioning. New York, Springer, 1996, pp 261–275.

10 Hudlicka O, Brown M, Egginton S: Angiogenesis in skeletal and cardiac muscle. Physiol Rev 1992;72:369–417.

11 Rakusan K, Cicutti N: The effect of acute and chronic hypoxia on coronary microcirculation. Hypoxia Med J 1996;4(3):3–7.

12 Rakusan K, Ehrenburg IV, Gulyaeva NV, Tkatchouk EN: The effect of intermittent normobaric hypoxia on myocardial structure in rats. Hypoxia Med J 1997;5(3):3–8.

13 Chen M, Zhou ZN: Effects of hypoxia on myoglobin and antioxidant enzymes in rat myocardium. Exp Clin Cardiol 1997;2(3):179–183.

14 Tse D, Zhou ZN: Effects of hypoxia on myoglobin in cultured rat myocytes (in Chinese). Sheng Li Hsueh Pao 1997;49:497–503.

15 McGrath JJ, Bullard RW: Altered myocardial performance in response to anoxia after high-altitude exposure. J Appl Physiol 1968;25:761–764.

16 Ziegelhoffer A, Prochazka J, Pelouch V, Ostadal B, Dzurba A, Vrbjar N: Increased affinity to substrate in sarcolemmal ATPases from hearts acclimatized to high-altitude hypoxia. Physiol Bohemoslov 1987;36:403–415.

17 Kopylov IuN, Golubeva LIu: Effect of adaptation to periodic hypoxia on the resistance of the indicators of energy metabolism and myocardial contraction in acute anoxia and reoxygenation. Biull Eksp Biol Med 1991;111(1):22–25.

18 Maher JT, Manchanda SC, Cymerman A, Wolfe DL, Hartley LH: Cardiovascular resonsiveness to beta-adrenergic stimulation and blockade in chronic hypoxia. Am J Physiol 1975;228:477–481.

19 Voelkel NF, Hegstrand L, Reeves JT, McMurty IF, Molinoff PB: Effects of hypoxia on density of β-adrenergic receptors. J Appl Physiol 1981;50:363–366.
20 Maher JT, Denniston JC, Wolfe DL: Mechanism of the attenuated cardiac response to beta-adrenergic stimulation in chronic hypoxia. J Appl Physiol 1978;44:647–651.
21 Faltova E, Mraz M, Pelouch V, Prochazka J, Ostadal B: Increase and regression of the protective effect of high-altitude acclimatization on the isoprenoline-induced necrotic lesions in the rat myocardium. Physiol Bohemoslov 1987;36:43–52.
22 Burtscher M, Tsvetkova AM, Tkatchouk EN, Brauchle G, Mitterbauer G, Gulyaeva NV, Kofler W: Effects of interval hypoxic training on cardiorespiratory respones to exercise. Hypoxia Med J 1997;5(3):13–14.
23 Lebedev AV, Sadretdinov SM, Pelouch V, Prochazka J, Levitsky DO, Ostadal B: Free radical membrane scavengers in myocardium of rats of different age exposed to chronic hypoxia. Biomed Biochim Acta 1989;48(2–3):S122–S125.
24 Meerson FZ: Adaptive Protection of the Heart. Moscow, CRC Press, 1991.
25 Iwaki K, Chi SH, Dillmann WH, Mestril R: Induction of HSP70 in cultured rat neonatal cardiomyocytes by hypoxia and metabolic stress. Circulation 1993;87:2023–2032.
26 Howard D, Geoghegan TE: Altered cardiac tissue gene expression during acute hypoxic exposure. Mol Cell Biochem 1986;69:155–160.
27 Meerson FZ, Malyshev IY, Zamotrinsky AV: Differences in adaptive stabilization of structures in responses to stress and hypoxia relate with the accumulation of hsp70 isoforms. Mol Cell Biochem 1992;111:87–95.
28 Katayose D, Isoyama S, Fujita H, Shibahara S: Separate regulation of heme oxygenase and heat shock protein 70 mRNA expression in the rat heart by hemodynamic stress. Biochem Biophys Res Commun 1993;191:587–594.
29 Parrat JR: Eicosanoids and arrhythmogenesis; in Vaughan-Williams EM (ed): Antiarrhythmic Drugs. Berlin, Springer, 1989, pp 569–589.
30 Karmazyn M, Dhalla NS: Physiological and pathophysiological aspects of cardiac prostaglandins. Can J Physiol Pharmacol 1983;61:1207–1225.
31 Richalet JP, Hornych A, Rathat C, Aumont J, Larmignat P, Remy P: Plasma prostaglandins, leukotrienes and thromboxane in acute high-altitude hypoxia. Respir Physiol 1991;85:205–215.
32 Pshennikova MG, Kuznetsova VA, Kopylov IuN, Shimkovich MV, Vovk VI, Saprygin DV, Meerson FZ: The role of the prostaglandin system in the cardioprotective effect of adaptation to hypoxia in stress (in Russian). Kardiologiia 1992;32:61–64.
33 Ziegelhoffer A, Grunermel J, Dzurba A, Prochazka J, Kolar F, Vrbjar N, Pelouch V, Ostadal B, Szeheres L: Sarcolemmal cation transport systems in rat hearts acclimatized to high-altitude hypoxia: Influence of 7-oxo-prostacyclin; in Ostadal B, Dhalla NS (eds): Heart Function in Health and Disease. Boston, Kluwer, 1992, pp 219–228.
34 Xu J, Tong H, Wang L, Hurt CM, Pelleg A: Endogenous adenosine, A_1 adenosine receptor, and pertussis-toxin-sensitive guanine nucleotide-binding protein mediate hypoxia induced AV nodal conduction block in guinea pig heart in vivo. Cardiovasc Res 1993;27:134–140.
35 Kacimi R, Richalet J-P, Crozatier B: Hypoxia-induced differnetial modulation of adenosinergic and muscarinic receptors in rat heart. J Appl Physiol 1993;75:1123–1128.
36 Parratt JR: Endogenous myocardial protective (antiarrhythmic) substances. Cardiovasc Res 1993:27:77–83.

Author Index Vol. 8, No. 4–5, 1999

Biological Signals and Receptors

KARGER
Fax + 41 61 306 12 34
E-Mail karger@karger.ch
www.karger.com

Accessible online at:
http://BioMedNet.com/karger

Subject Index Vol. 8, No. 4–5, 1999

Biological Signals and Receptors

KARGER

Fax + 41 61 306 12 34
E-Mail karger@karger.ch
www.karger.com

Accessible online at:
http://BioMedNet.com/karger

Cross-talk between the immune and neuroendocrine systems

Neuroendocrine Control of the Thymus

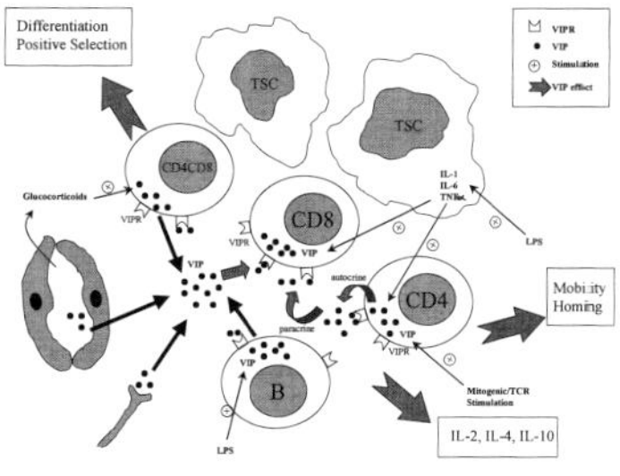

Editor: W. Savino

The thymus, which plays a vital role in the control of the immune system, is looked at from different angles such as the immune-neuroendocrine network from development to aging, the selection process of developing T cells, and the interdependence of the neuroendocrine and immune systems and their communication circuitries.

The information compiled in this issue will allow immunologists in general, in particular those working in thymus physiology and/or pathology, to take into account the hormones, neuropeptides and neurotransmitters that are relevant in various aspects comprised in the physiology of the thymus.

Endocrinologists and neurobiologists who work at the interface with the immune system will find a wealth of new information, since many of the concepts discussed in relation to the thymus can be extrapolated to immunoneuroendocrine interactions occurring in the periphery.

Contents

Neuroimmunomodulation
Editors: McCann, S.M. (Dallas, Tex.); Lipton, J.M. (Dallas, Tex.)
ISSN 1021–7401
Hard cover reprint: Vol. 6, No. 1–2 (1999)

Neuroendocrine Control of the Thymus
Editor: Savino, W. (Rio de Janeiro)
144 p., 33 fig., 4 in color, 18 tab., hard cover, 1999
CHF 52.– / DEM 62.– / USD 45.25
Prices subject to change
DEM price for Germany, USD price for USA only
ISBN 3–8055–6769–3

Fields of Interest: Neurology; Immunology; Neuroendocrinology

KI 99423

KARGER